The Missing Diagnosis II

C. Orian Truss, M.D.

Published by

C. Orian Truss, M.D.
2614 Highland Avenue
Birmingham, Alabama 35205

***

First Printing April 2009

***

Orders for additional copies of this book may be sent to the following address:

C. Orian Truss, M.D.
2614 Highland Avenue
Birmingham, Alabama 35205

ISBN: 978-0-615-27396-9

Dedication

There are many ways in which family members play an important role in whatever one is attempting, but none more important than their continuing interest in your progress. This is particularly important when inevitable snags occur and progress halts. This is my acknowledgment to them for their participation in this work that has spanned many years.

My wife Susan for her ever-present patience, encouragement, and pride in this work that covered 56 years.

Our 5 wonderful children: Christopher, Tommy, Julie, Johnny, and Sally.

Our 14 grandchildren:

Anna Truss Ostrom
Wiley Dewitt Truss
Susan Todd Truss
Alex Turner Truss
Lucy Childs Olson
Elizabeth Ann Childs
George Thomas Childs
Ivan Orian Smith Truss
Michael John Truss
Mary Catherine Truss
Thomas Young Jordan
Susanna Jordan Brown
Mary Kate Jordan
Polly Rebecca Jordan

Four "very new" great-grandchildren:

Jane Frances Ostrom
Charles Phillip Olson
Elisabeth Brittain Olson
Charles Wheeler Brown

Special Acknowledgment

On occasion there arises a need to come up with just the right words to express adequately one's admiration and gratitude for the many ways in which one's job has been made easier by a particular individual.

Such is the case now as I recall the hiring of a part time employee for my medical practice. Kenny Lenoir had returned to college in preparation for a teaching career. Little did I know what I was getting when I hired this young man!

Now, 25 years later, it seems impossible to find words that adequately express Kenny's numerous skills that accompany his genuine compassion for the chronically ill people with whom we have dealt on a daily basis.

That the patients, in turn, sensed and appreciated his concern is shown best in that I have had not a single complaint in these 25 years.

Therefore, may I conclude by saying, for each patient and for myself,

Thank you Kenny

Acknowledgments

Shirley Tatum – For 25 years Shirley was not just my bookkeeper but also the "mother" of the office staff, tending to any problem that arose during the many busy days that she was with us.

Lillie Jordan – Since the late 1970s this wonderful Christian lady has been not so much an employee, but a part of our family. Without her close care for the past six years, I could not have continued. Everyone who has benefited from my care may thank her.

Juanita Clouse – Her help with secretarial duties, insurance, and the many day-to-day concerns that arise in patient care were of great value.

Barbara Dickey – Barbara headed our research laboratory, but even before that, helped greatly with library work, even before funding was available.

Carol Lowe – Carol was of great help in our laboratory studies. She contributed greatly to these later studies.

Very special thanks to Lauren Graffeo for her expert help with statistics and graphing.

Special thanks to Sue Smith for her time and editing expertise.

And to the many other workers and patients who helped by participating in these studies, both as subjects as well as by their encouragement as the studies progressed.

Dr. Truss is a graduate of Birmingham-Southern College and of Cornell University Medical College. His post-graduate training was on the Cornell Division of Bellevue Hospital in New York City, where he completed successive years as Intern, Assistant Resident, and Chief Resident in Internal Medicine. He later held the positions of Chief of Cardiology and Assistant Chief of Medicine at the U. S. Air Force Hospital at Maxwell Field, Alabama. There followed a year devoted to study of the female endocrine system as a Fellow in Pharmacology at the University of Alabama Medical College in Birmingham.

Dr. Truss served as Instructor in Medicine at Cornell Medical College and as Instructor in Clinical Medicine at the University of Alabama Medical College prior to devoting full time to private practice. Dr. Truss is a certified specialist (Diplomate) of the American Board of Internal Medicine and a member of numerous medical organizations.

For many years his private practice has focused on the relationship of allergy and infection to many of the problems dealt with by internists. In particular, this interest has centered on the role of the yeast "Candida albicans" in human illness.

The Missing Diagnosis, first published in 1983, is a book about human illness caused by the yeast "Candida albicans." It covers the first 22 years of Dr. Truss' interest in the varied clinical symptoms that may be associated with allergic or toxic responses to products of Candida albicans, as well as the more familiar ones originating at the sites of yeast growth in the body. *The Missing Diagnosis II* presents Dr. Truss' observations over the last 25 years on the diagnosis and treatment of chronic yeast infections. Both books have been written especially for the patient.

CONTENTS

PART THREE:

SCIENTIFIC

PREFACE*

Present in all of us, at birth or soon thereafter, is a fungus that lives primarily on the skin, in the gastrointestinal tract, and in women in the vagina. Its name is Candida albicans. It is considered a member of the "normal flora" that live on these body surfaces. A number of familiar conditions occur when this yeast infects these surfaces—diaper rash, oral thrush, "athlete's foot," "jock itch," nail infections, vaginitis, etc. It has not been considered the cause of other "generalized" symptoms—merely the "local" symptoms at the sites of infections, e.g., the vagina, between the toes, etc. These infections of the body surfaces are known as "superficial candidiasis."

Careful attention to the patient's history, however, often reveals the presence of a number of other symptoms that had begun soon after the appearance of the local symptoms. These include loss of energy, inappropriate depression, impairment of short-term memory and concentration, menstrual problems, decreased libido, impotence, premenstrual tension, and other symptoms previously reported. *By listening to the patient*, it is possible to identify a number of symptoms that began as the local symptoms became chronic, and that disappeared as the local symptoms were brought under control. Listen to the patient!!

It is now 25 years since publication of *The Missing Diagnosis*, the book that told of the first 22 years of my interest in chronic symptoms related to the yeast "Candida albicans"—a fungus present in all of us, essentially from birth until death, as evidenced by the presence in everyone of bloodstream antibodies to this organism.

In a series of papers that I feel were of great importance, it was reported that in pooled human blood from healthy individuals, 79 antibodies had been found that reacted in the laboratory with Candida albicans, thus identifying this yeast as the source of 79 different substances ("antigens"), each of which had stimulated formation of its own antibody. (Each antibody will react only with the antigen that stimulated its formation. As an example, an antibody formed in

*This publication is intended primarily for patients. Therefore references will not be republished but may be found in previous publications. Also a number of terms will be clarified (parenthetically) for the non-professional reader—"the patient."

response to a "flu shot" reacts only with the influenza virus, the "antigen.")

While these 79 antibodies reacted in a test tube with Candida albicans, thus identifying this fungus as the source of the 79 foreign substances that had stimulated their formation, this does not identify these antigens—only that they came from Candida albicans. The concept that led to this knowledge was, in my opinion, brilliant and points to the probable source of the many generalized symptoms that often accompany chronic superficial yeast infections. The identification of these yeast-derived antigens, and of the mechanism by which they disturb normal physiologic processes, is a promising field for future research.

Yeast had attracted little attention prior to three major developments in the practice of medicine. From 1900 to the mid-1930s the Index Medicus listed only a dozen or so papers published annually under the heading "Monilia albicans" and later "Candida albicans." This changed abruptly in 1936 with the first of three valuable additions to medical practice—antibacterial therapy. With the availability of penicillin as the war ended, and particularly with the beginning of "broad-spectrum" antibiotic availability in 1947 (aureomycin), the incidence of yeast infections continued to rise. Further, the highly dangerous "systemic candidiasis" was reported, wherein yeast spreads through the bloodstream to infect one or more internal organs.*

To make matters worse, as far as yeast is concerned, in 1950 cortisone was discovered. This led to a further explosion of reports of yeast vaginitis in the same percentage (35%) of women as had been estimated to have been caused by antibiotics. But most importantly, this also led to immunosuppression as a treatment option in an ever increasing number of conditions.

Soon thereafter the "birth control pill" added its impact to the stimulation of this yeast, now known as Candida albicans, but which had gone through many name changes since its discovery well over a century earlier. During the span of time that encompassed the absorption into medical practice of these three major modalities of treatment,

*"Systemic" or "deep" candidiasis almost always is seen when a patient's immunity is extremely low, e.g., HIV, leukemia, lymphoma, or when therapeutic immunosuppression has been employed.

the increase in incidence of acute yeast vaginitis has been estimated to approach 1500%, with the percentage of cases of acute vaginitis caused by yeast increasing from 25% in 1940 to 90% in 1965.

The advent of broad-spectrum antibiotic therapy also marked the beginning of my interest in Candida albicans. At the time that I was serving as Chief Resident on the Cornell Medical College Division of Bellevue Hospital, I was charged with overseeing the supply of terramycin provided for pre-release testing in the treatment of lobar pneumonia. (The capsules were selling on the "black market" for several dollars each.) We were told to use 1,000 mg every 4 hours "around the clock." This proved to be two to four times the eventual dose.

I learned very early in my career about the relation of antibiotics to yeast infections. In addition to the familiar vaginal symptoms of itching and discharge, yeast overgrowth often occurs also in the colon, leading to excess gas and bloating, accompanied by constipation or diarrhea, and possibly rectal itching.

Today, after appropriate work-up returns only normal results, these G.I. symptoms are almost always correctly diagnosed as IBS (irritable bowel syndrome) but mistakenly attributed to "stress." Nystatin, an anti-fungal drug, in the proper dose alleviates these symptoms, thus identifying their true cause.

Four years later an event was to occur that demonstrated convincingly how Candida albicans was being ignored as a significant factor in human illness. This case is described in detail later in this report. Briefly, in 1953 a coal miner was given the antibiotic aureomycin when a cut finger became infected. Immediate diarrhea was followed by fever, cough, marked weight loss, and 6 months hospitalization. Treatment with cortisone, antibiotics, and many other drugs failed to slow the progressive downhill course.

Detailed examination of the massive (6 month) hospital chart revealed that two sputum cultures had been positive for Candida albicans. This was ignored by the many consultants who had been involved in the case; it was considered an "opportunistic" infection of a patient who was dying from an as yet undiagnosed disease. When requestioning revealed how the illness had begun—diarrhea from aureomycin given for an infected finger—treatment of this yeast led to a full recovery.

The final stimulus to my interest in Candida albicans arose when one of my children developed severe asthma, leading eventually to my adding the treatment of allergies to my practice of Internal Medicine. Four years later it became necessary that I limit my practice to allergies. It was at this point that the importance of yeast in human illness could be explored in depth, resulting eventually in the publication of 5 papers and a book detailing my experiences and conclusions regarding the importance of Candida albicans in human health. The first paper, "Tissue Injury Induced by Candida Albicans: Mental and Neurologic Manifestations," was presented after 16 years of investigation. My book—*The Missing Diagnosis*—was published 6 years later.

The present book—*The Missing Diagnosis II*—is a sequel to the first; it represents the most recent 25 years of observations in diagnosing and treating chronic yeast infections.

While one purpose of the present book is to update the views expressed in the earlier publications, a primary purpose also is to present for patients an informal discussion as to how they may conduct a "therapeutic trial" to see if this may be the answer to frustrating health problems that have defied the many attempts to elucidate their cause. Patients carrying out such a diagnostic therapeutic trial will find interesting the results of studies of carbohydrate handling in a group of women with symptoms essentially identical to theirs. Published herein as my 6th paper, it is titled, "Membrane Transport in Patients with Chronic Superficial Yeast Infections: Insulin Resistance and Glycosuria—The Metabolic Syndrome."

This 6th paper shows strikingly consistent abnormalities in carbohydrate handling in 52 women with symptoms of the "superficial candidiasis syndrome" (SCS).* When the yeast infection is properly treated, the simultaneous disappearance of the generalized symptoms as the local symptoms are brought under control, together with return to normal of the pretreatment laboratory abnormalities in carbohydrate handling (impaired glucose tolerance, insulin resistance, etc.), establishes the relation of these symptoms to these metabolic abnormalities, and of both to the partial, temporary loss of control of Candida albicans.

*The "superficial candidiasis syndrome" is the term that I use when generalized symptoms accompany the local symptoms at the sites of skin and mucous membrane infections. "Superficial candidiasis" is the designation when only local symptoms are present.

I emphasize the fact that these publications present my personal experiences and beliefs regarding Candida albicans. “My doctor says that he (she) doesn’t believe in chronic candidiasis” is a statement that many patients have relayed to me. The latest textbooks continue to treat yeast as more of a nuisance than as a significant cause of chronic ill health, the principal exception being the instances of deep (formerly “systemic”) candidiasis associated primarily with diseases of the cells of the immune system itself (HIV, leukemia, lymphoma, etc.).

When something new is reported in medicine, normally others try to duplicate it. To the best of my knowledge, there have been no such papers published. Many have expressed their disbelief, but not because of a failure to confirm.

Finally, it is important to stress that the “therapeutic trial” is for diagnosis rather than treatment. Patients should consult their physicians regarding long-term dietary changes since other conditions may be affected adversely. Further, since the diet is just one of the components of treatment, it alone cannot be expected to bring this fungus infection under control.

If the three to six weeks trial of a low carbohydrate-low yeast diet results in partial or total relief of a number of the characteristic symptoms of the “superficial candidiasis syndrome” (SCS), treatment should be placed in the hands of the patient’s physician or another physician, preferrably one trained in treating allergies.

The diet used to point to this diagnosis may need to be modified to take into consideration other medical problems that may be present. Also, the diet requires adjustment as improvement continues. For these reasons a physician is essential to supervise long-term treatment.

The usual way of presenting graphs and tables (when articles are published in medical journals) is to include each one in the text on the same or a facing page. In this instance we are presenting them together at the end of the text. This method was chosen because in a number of instances the same graph is referred to in several places in the text; rather than duplicating a graph each time it is referenced, the page number will be listed in the text.

Finally, the book is divided into three parts. Part One is for the patient’s use in understanding and possibly carrying out several simple diagnostic tests that include variations in diet in a search for evidence that Candida albicans is out of control—a “therapeutic trial.” True food allergies must be ruled out when diet affects symptoms; this too is discussed.

Part Two is a general discussion of a variety of factors related to the diagnosis and treatment of SCS. This section should be of interest to patients and physicians alike. It includes some conditions not previously reported as yeast-related.

Part Three is the "SCIENTIFIC" section, containing a new (6th) paper not previously published. Also in this section is speculation and ideas for future research into this subject.

Appendix I: Included in this section is a long-term follow-up of several patients presented in my first book (*The Missing Diagnosis*, 1983); the page number (from the softcover edition) is shown for each case. These are included as reassurances that relapse was highly unlikely once these very ill patients had regained their health.

Appendix II: In my first book, the three papers published prior to the book were reprinted with appropriate page references. In the current book—*The Missing Diagnosis II*—the 4th and 5th papers are reprinted in this section, while the 6th paper is published (for the first time) in the text of the book (Part Three).

PART ONE

BACKGROUND AND DIAGNOSIS

Chapter 1
Background and Present Concepts

Background: My interest in Candida albicans—an interest that was to last for almost 6 decades—began quite by accident. Because at the time I was Chief Resident in Internal Medicine on the Cornell Division of Bellevue Hospital, I was given the responsibility of safeguarding a large supply of broad-spectrum antibiotics* supplied to Cornell for pre-marketing testing in the treatment of lobar pneumonia. We were told to use 1,000 mg every 4 hours "around the clock"—some 2 to 4 times the eventual dose. I learned early in my career that broad-spectrum antibiotics stir up yeast vaginitis and diarrhea!

My next encounter with Candida albicans occurred some 4 years later when for 2 weeks I covered the practice of a leading internist, prior to opening my own office. This case, alluded to in "Preface," is now presented in greater detail. A 45-year-old man was near death after 6 months of hospitalization. High, spiking fever coincided with a productive cough and infiltrate throughout the lungs, with pericardial effusion, and with 40 lb. weight loss. Two sputum cultures had been positive for Candida albicans but, as usual, this was considered "secondary" to whatever the primary illness happened to be. However, requestioning revealed that six months earlier this man had been in perfect health, working as a coal miner, when he cut a finger that soon became infected. Aureomycin led to immediate and severe diarrhea. Fever and cough led to hospitalization and treatment with numerous antibiotics as well as steroids and other immunosuppressants—all to no avail. A library search yielded a report of 2 cases of "systemic candidiasis" that had recovered when treated with saturated solution of potassium iodide—a drug that we had used extensively as an expectorant during house-staff training. This led to immediate improvement and eventual lasting recovery. This case reinforced my earlier experience with broad-spectrum antibiotics and diarrhea, except that in this instance the

*At this time these were selling on the "black market" for $4-5 per capsule.

yeast spread rapidly to many internal organs, almost costing a man his life.

My final and lasting interest in Candida albicans occurred after I had added the treatment of allergies to my practice of internal medicine. Briefly, a 41-year-old woman, already being treated for nasal and sinus allergy, walked into the office with severe premenstrual depression and a severe migraine headache. Also present was a flare-up of yeast vaginitis. Using a technique that sometimes helps identify the cause of an allergic symptom, and on the hypothesis that perhaps an allergic reaction to yeast products was causing the migraine headache and severe depression, an extremely dilute dose of yeast extract was administered subcutaneously. Within 20 minutes both the depression and the headache had completely cleared. These symptoms had recurred by the next day and again were quickly relieved by the yeast extract. Sixteen years later these and subsequent experiences with Candida albicans were published in the first* of 5 papers, and subsequently in a book—*The Missing Diagnosis.***

This present book also contains a previously unpublished (6th) paper— "Membrane Transport in Patients with Chronic Superficial Yeast Infections: Insulin Resistance, Glycosuria, and the Metabolic Syndrome." This 6th paper presents detailed studies of carbohydrate metabolism before and during treatment in women with chronic yeast infections. Presented is evidence for the presence of abnormalities in membrane function, and for the presence of "insulin resistance" and "the metabolic syndrome." Each of these abnormalities in blood and urine resolves coincidentally with clearing of the presenting symptoms, both "local" and "generalized," that had accompanied the chronic yeast infections.

<u>Trends in Candida albicans</u>: Following this brief background to my continuing interest in Candida albicans and its relation to human health problems, we will consider certain "trends" that

---

*Truss, C. O. Tissue injury induced by Candida albicans: mental and neurologic manifestations. J. Orthomolecular Psychiatry 1978; 7: 17-37.

** Truss, C. O. *The Missing Diagnosis*, 1st Ed. Birmingham, AL. The Missing Diagnosis, Inc. 1983.

have paralleled the trend in yeast infections and that may be related, although in as yet unrecognized ways.

Considering possible relationships among such trends in the incidence and behavior of various diseases may be important and helpful, but they also may be easily overlooked. Despite the difficulty in determining cause and effect, simply considering the possibility of such relationships may point the way to important avenues of investigation into the etiologies (causes) of the many diseases that as yet have defied elucidation.

The first trend that has been well-documented is the progressive increase in the incidence of vaginal yeast infections following the introduction of antibacterial drugs in 1935. Vaginitis is used in most studies of the incidence of yeast infections, primarily because of the ready availability of vaginal secretions for diagnostic identification. It is important to recall, however, that the same is often occurring in the G.I. tract as one or more of several symptoms—gas/bloating, constipation/diarrhea, rectal itching, and indigestion/reflux. Except for the indigestion/reflux, these symptoms are almost always diagnosed as "irritable bowel syndrome" and are usually mistakenly attributed to "stress." In 1940 it was estimated that approximately 25 of every 100 cases of acute vaginitis were due to yeast, with 75 due primarily to Trichomonas, an unrelated organism. By 1965, 90 of every 100 cases were caused by Candida albicans. Stated differently, it has been estimated that there had been a 1500% increase in the incidence of acute vaginitis caused by yeast—an increase that began with the introduction of antibiotics into medical practice, followed soon thereafter by further increases in incidence related to the discovery of steroids and contraceptive hormones, and finally to the ever-increasing practice of suppressing the immune system as the primary treatment of many diseases.

It is also significant that the dangerous and often fatal dissemination of Candida albicans to internal organs had never been described until 1939. This condition, known then as "systemic candidiasis" (more recently as "deep candidiasis") has assumed ever-increasing importance over the subsequent decades, often being the terminal event in diseases of the cells of the immune system itself (white blood cells). Leukemia and HIV infections are such diseases where the loss of immune function is so severe that yeast often spreads through the bloodstream to multiple internal organs. Such "deep candidiasis" is difficult to diagnose and treat; it is rarely a threat in the absence of these diseases of the white blood cells themselves.

One major trend (noted above) that undoubtedly has added to the problem of loss of immunologic control of Candida albicans is the widespread adoption of deliberate immunosuppression as a way of treating numerous chronic conditions, particularly those diseases that are designated as "autoimmune." As treatment, the entire immune system is unavoidably weakened in order to weaken the immunologic attack on the patient's own organ (or organs). Even when this approach helps the symptoms in question, overgrowth of Candida albicans will almost certainly result to some degree, particularly when coupled with recurring courses of antibiotics and steroids.

During these same years, in work that I feel was of great significance, a series of papers was published reporting that pooled human blood from healthy individuals had been found to contain 79 antibodies that reacted in the laboratory with Candida albicans, an estimated 30-40 of the 79 antibodies being present in a single individual.* Since an antibody reacts specifically with the foreign substance (the "antigen") that stimulated the immune system to generate the antibody, we are forced to conclude that there is a total of 79 substances fed into the human bloodstream by this universally present yeast (a "fungus" or "mold"). Stated differently, even though these 79 antigens have not themselves been identified, the reaction of each of the 79 antibodies with Candida albicans identifies this yeast as the source of each of the foreign substances that had triggered these antibody responses by the human immune system.

It isn't clear whether the number and quantity of these anti-candida antibodies were increasing—i.e., whether this was a "trend"—or whether the constant increase in the number reported merely represented more sensitive laboratory techniques, so that antibodies were now being found that were missed in the earlier studies. In fact, both processes might well be responsible. It would seem that the former would be expected in view of the

---

*Axelson, Kirkpatrick and Buckley.: Scand. J. Immunol. Vol. 5, 177-190, 1976.

enormous increase in the incidence of chronic yeast infections; an accompanying increase in the release of these antigens would be expected to occur.

Isolated reports have been published of allergic reactions to yeast, based on the observation that common allergic conditions (e.g., asthma, migraine headaches, chronic urticaria) ceased with clearing of the yeast infection. Also, depression of the human immune system by Candida albicans itself has been reported and has been designated "immunologic paralysis" or "immunologic tolerance."* Other than such allergic symptoms, and this weakening of the immune system, the effect of these antigens or antibodies on human biochemistry or physiology is unknown. It would seem that this is truly a fertile field for investigation by the many sophisticated laboratory techniques now available.

Trends in other diseases: We turn now to trends that have occurred with respect to other diseases and symptoms, repeating for *emphasis* this well known fact: the more or less simultaneous occurrence of two things does *not* constitute proof that one is the cause of the other.

But neither can we exclude the *possibility* that the two trends are somehow related, particularly in an etiological (causative) way. Recognition of such a relationship, if it exists, may lead to additional studies that will help our understanding of either or both conditions.

We have already seen the tremendous increase in yeast infections over the last six decades, beginning with the introduction of antibiotics and soon thereafter of steroids and "birth control pills." Paralleling this increase in the incidence of yeast infections is the indisputable increase in the incidence of Type II ("adult onset") diabetes mellitus. The demonstration in patients with SCS, reported in the new paper in this book, of insulin resistance that clears with anti-yeast treatment is highly relevant. Type II diabetes is a condition characterized by abnormally high blood sugar (glucose) levels despite levels of blood insulin that are higher than normal, at least in the beginning. This is known as "insulin resistance." By convention, diabetes is diagnosed when,

*References 1-9 in the bibliography of the new paper presented elsewhere in this book.

on a 2-hour glucose tolerance test, either the fasting blood glucose *or* the blood sugar at 2 hours is elevated to a certain agreed upon level. Reference to the graph on page 119 (fig. 2) of this book shows the consistency of insulin resistance in 52* patients, based on a pretreatment 2-hour glucose tolerance test; it also shows the range of the severity of this insulin resistance, up to and including true diabetes (Case One—page 120 fig. 3).

The mechanism by which Candida albicans is inducing insulin resistance is not clear. The membrane abnormalities reported in 1984** and in the current paper might well be important in view of the many reported defects in enzyme and receptor function already reported to be associated with increased membrane rigidity (see current paper for literature review).

Acetaldehyde and carbon dioxide are products of fermentation of glucose by yeast. Acetaldehyde is a highly reactive substance that can alter membrane rigidity. In our studies it was frequently found both in breath and in erythrocytes (red blood cells); the laboratory technique used was gas chromatography.

The acetaldehyde studies will be made the subject of a separate report. Briefly, varying amounts would be present at any time of day or night, either when fasting or after eating. For example, acetaldehyde might be abundant in the breath at 7:00 a.m. and absent when measured 3-4 hours later (or vice versa). Efforts to force its appearance by feeding a high carbohydrate meal were unsuccessful. When measured repeatedly in the same patient over several days, it could reappear in the breath at any time, as though it were building up and then "blowing off."

Acetaldehyde binds avidly to proteins at what are termed "sulfhydryl" and "amine" sites on the protein. It has been studied extensively by researchers in the field of alcoholism, since conversion of alcohol to acetaldehyde, primarily in the liver, is the first major step as the body rids itself of alcohol.

---

*Of the 53 patients studied, "peak insulin" was available in only 52 patients because of difficulty with venopuncture in the remaining subject.

**Truss, C. O. Metabolic abnormalities in patients with chronic candidiasis: the acetaldehyde hypothesis. J. Orthomolecular Psychiatry 1984: 13: 66-93.

This brings us to another theoretical mechanism by which Candida albicans could be causing insulin resistance. As acetaldehyde is produced in the gastrointestinal tract (fermentation of glucose by Candida albicans), it is absorbed into what is known as the "portal circulation," by which it is carried into the liver.

This is highly significant. Insulin, which is a protein, is released into the portal blood, whereas most hormones enter the systemic circulation. Since insulin is a protein, and since it is released by the pancreas directly into the portal circulation, it will be in contact with acetaldehyde, should this highly reactive substance have entered the portal circulation by absorption from the G.I. tract after having been formed there by fermentation of glucose by Candida albicans. It is hard to believe that the function of an insulin molecule would not be impaired should acetaldehyde bind to multiple amine and sulfhydral sites on the newly formed insulin molecule.

Thus, if it can be demonstrated that the *function* of the newly released insulin molecules has been immediately impaired by portal blood acetaldehyde binding to its amine groups (Schiff bases) or its sulfhydryl groups (thiols), the insulin resistance would have been explained.

Ideally, portal blood would be sampled, but this is not feasible in humans. Insulin in peripheral blood should, however, still be abnormal if these reactions had occurred in portal blood. Impaired function of insulin, such that more insulin than normal is required to attain a given level of blood sugar, actually defines "insulin resistance."

Other proteins (e.g., serum proteins) circulating in portal blood would likewise be modified by similar acetaldehyde binding. In patients with SCS, many abnormalities were found in proteins and fats (previously reported).*

The "obesity epidemic" is the subject of almost daily articles in the media as well as in the medical journals. Many other diseases have been reported to have increased in incidence. Examples (in addition to Type II diabetes and obesity) include

---

*Truss, C. O. Metabolic abnormalities in patients with chronic candidiasis: the acetaldehyde hypothesis. J. Orthomolecular Psychiatry 1984: 13: 66-93.

asthma, "lupus," and anorexia nervosa. As stated earlier, it is difficult to determine whether what seems to be an increase in incidence is actually due, at least partially, to better diagnosis.

In most patients who have regained their health with anti-yeast treatment, often after many years of symptoms, a variety of diagnoses had been entertained. Common examples are "lupus," rheumatoid arthritis, the "chronic fatigue syndrome" and "fibromyalgia," the "irritable bowel syndrome" (IBS), and gastroesophageal reflux disease (GERD).

In fact, many of these "diagnoses" merely represent the current practice of designating as a "disease" what heretofore had been merely a symptom: fatigue (chronic fatigue syndrome), muscle/joint pain (fibromyalgia), diarrhea/constipation/gas/bloating (IBS, or irritable bowel syndrome), depression ("Clinical depression"), etc. However, it is my opinion that giving a symptom a new name and calling it a new "disease" is not justified merely because we can't find the cause of the symptom.

My first paper,* and subsequently my book, reported the individual symptoms associated with partial loss of immunologic control of Candida albicans. In a more recent paper these symptoms were compared to the symptoms of the "chronic fatigue syndrome," as reported in the initial paper defining this "new disease"; they were found to be identical (Table 1).** Further, the symptoms of "fibromyalgia" and "chronic fatigue syndrome" are so similar that many believe these to be the same condition. In any event, these are symptoms that often clear with proper anti-yeast therapy.

Finally, the prominent symptom of difficulty with short-term memory and concentration has led to a variety of diagnoses, with suitable acronyms, that relegate the patient to the psychosomatic category and engender the admonition that "stress" is the underlying cause of the problem.

---

*Truss, C.O. Tissue injury induced by candida albicans: mental and neurologic manifestations. J Orthomolecular Psychiatry 1978; 7: 17-37.

**Truss, C.O. Generalized symptoms in women with chronic yeast vaginitis. J. Advancement in Medicine 1992; 5: 139-175.

"Stress" is indeed present in everyone throughout life, thus providing a convenient explanation of symptoms and diseases despite the total lack of evidence that "stress" is related to the symptoms. But Candida albicans too is present in everyone throughout life, feeding into the bloodstream varying amounts of foreign proteins and probably acetaldehyde. The amount of acetaldehyde would be expected to vary with the degree of yeast overgrowth at a given time, this in turn being affected by a high glucose (carbohydrate) diet, antibiotics, "birth control pills," steroids, therapeutic immunosuppression, and probably the patient's genetic makeup as it influences immunologic responses to different strains of yeast.

In children the favorite designation for this abnormality of brain function is "ADHD"—"attention deficit hyperactivity disorder." (Children cannot be expected to use the same words as adults would use in describing such symptoms.) More recently "ADD" ("attention deficit disorder") has gained favor in adults with difficulty concentrating. Again, "stress" is almost always invoked when the diagnostician is pressed for an answer as to the *cause* of the problem.

This remains true even though the patient protests that there is no significant stress present. Even when stress is present, the assumption is not justified that "stress" is the cause of the symptoms. However, since "stress" is present in everyone throughout life, it is unnecessary to "prove" its presence; it provides a ready answer when the physician is pressed for the "cause" of the symptoms. Further, to the patient it is a much better accepted term than "hypochondriac" or "psychosomatic."

The great disadvantage to *either* term is that it virtually guarantees the cessation of further efforts to uncover the true cause of the chronic symptoms. The patient has been relegated to the "psychosomatic" category.

New "diseases": There seems to be no end to the practice of designating a symptom as a new "disease," most often attributing it to "stress" and prescribing accordingly. As stated above, the "chronic fatigue syndrome," "fibromyalgia," "Clinical depression," "irritable bowel syndrome" (IBS), "attention deficit hyperactivity disorder" (ADHD), or in adults "attention deficit disorder" (ADD), "gastroesophageal reflux disease" (GERD), etc., etc., are all good examples of this practice.

I suppose no harm would follow except that, when asked for the cause of the symptoms, the reflex answer "stress" is invoked. At that point, in the physician's mind the problem has been solved—the cause of the condition has been found and treatment begun. Unfortunately, many of the drugs chosen may be toxic or addictive, and the patient may be on them for years. Most important is the frequent discontinuing of the search for the true cause of the chronic symptoms once the physician has attributed them to "stress."

Two examples illustrate this sequence of events. The first is the demonstration that peptic ulcers are due to the bacterium H. pylori, *not* to "stress" as had been the accepted cause for many decades. The second illustration is a symptom that is perhaps the most characteristic of all the symptoms that cease when Candida albicans is brought under control. This is the distressing symptom of marked impairment of short-term memory and of concentration. To term this "ADD" is to assure that the wrong treatment will be instituted.

It is important to keep searching for the true cause of symptoms rather than to embark on a course of treatment based on the assumption that we are dealing with a "stand-alone" disease caused by stress. Only because someone was not willing to accept this assumption are we now treating peptic ulcers with antibiotics.

Chapter 2
When to Suspect Candida albicans

When a woman has chronic intractable yeast vaginitis with G.I. tract symptoms, the diagnosis is very simple. When to suspect this diagnosis if no such vaginal or intestinal symptoms are present is another (and very important) matter. This is illustrated by the following case:

A previously healthy 66-year-old man developed asthma 5 years before his initial visit to me. He came with the complaints of 3 years of chronic intestinal discomfort associated with alternating diarrhea/constipation, and much gas and bloating. The asthma had reached the severity that limited his walking to "half a block."

One year before his first visit to me, he had a thorough investigation by a gastroenterologist in a major teaching hospital; no abnormality was found and no diagnosis was made.

An additional mysterious finding was a strange tumor on the skin at elbow level of one arm. It was 2 inches in length, raised and very firm, and purple in color. Over the 7 years of its presence, this tumor had been unchanging. It had been biopsied 3 times; in each case the pathologist's diagnosis was leukemia or SLE (systemic lupus erythematosis).

Within 24 hours of beginning nystatin therapy (4 tablets 4 times daily) and appropriate diet, the G.I. symptoms were gone! At the end of the first week of therapy, his words were "my asthma is 75% gone." At 10 days the strange tumor—a tumor that had been unchanging for 7 years—had softened and become lighter in color. At 10 weeks it had disappeared without a scar. The skin was entirely normal!

Thus, the "generalized" manifestations of asthma and the tumor had their onset 2 years and 4 years respectively *before* the colon symptoms. In other words, the site of the yeast infection in the colon was *symptomatically silent* during the first 4 years of the tumor's presence. Only after the tumor had been present for 4 years, and the asthma for 2 years, did the yeast infection in the colon affect the function of this organ, leading to the distressing colon symptoms for which he was seeking help. Had I seen him 3 years earlier, there would have been *nothing* to suggest a yeast infection. The "local" symptoms appeared 4 years *after* the first generalized symptom!

Thus is established a very important principle. This diagnosis may be entertained even while the local yeast infection (in this case, in the colon) is still symptomatically silent. Yeast products were in this case already inducing symptoms at sites distant to the site where yeast had penetrated the mucous membrane of the colon to gain access to the bloodstream. Such access to the bloodstream, occurring as it did for several years prior to the onset of IBS symptoms, allowed generalized symptoms to be induced even though local symptoms were still absent. The yeast infection itself remained silent; for 4 years (the tumor) and 2 years (the asthma) there was nothing to suggest yeast as the cause of these generalized symptoms.

At this time I know of no way to diagnose such yeast-induced generalized symptoms, other than a brief therapeutic trial of an anti-yeast drug and suitable diet. We may anticipate advances in knowledge that will someday identify the earliest biochemical changes induced by such antigenic substances being released by this yeast. Such biochemical changes, if measurable, should provide a suitable test for such subtle yeast effects in humans.

Conclusion: Of the greatest importance is the principle illustrated by this case. Armed with the knowledge that 1) yeast, usually Candida albicans, is in everyone and 2) anti-Candida antibodies have been demonstrated in all of us, we are forced to conclude that the yeast antigens responsible for the formation of these antibodies (or indeed the antibodies themselves) may be inducing generalized symptoms *long before* the appearance of the classical symptoms we associate with the *local* tissue invasion of the yeast itself (e.g., vaginal itching and discharge, "athlete's foot," "IBS," thrush, etc.). Symptoms that clear with appropriate yeast suppression will require that we think of this fungus as the cause of illnesses that heretofore we have not connected with yeast.

Chapter 3
My Approach to the Diagnosis of SCS (Superficial Candidiasis Syndrome)

Part One of this book is primarily for patients. Its purpose is, by describing in detail my approach to the diagnosis, treatment, and prevention of illness resulting from chronic tissue penetration by the yeast "Candida albicans," to help patients evaluate this as the possible cause of their chronic symptoms.

Each week at 8:00 a.m. I sit across the desk from another in a seemingly endless parade of young women* with the same chronic complaints, and the same frustration at the inability of the medical profession to find their cause. In today's sophisticated diagnostic environment, the inability to find their cause virtually guarantees that these multi-system complaints will have repeatedly been attributed to "stress." This in turn leads to symptomatic drug treatment rather than to treatment that attacks the cause of these symptoms. Eventually many of these patients turn to the health food store and to "alternate" drugs, their cost and possible side effects only adding to the problem.

Diet will form the central theme of this discussion, first how it may aggravate yeast infections, then how its manipulation aids in arriving at the correct diagnosis. We will suggest ways in which patients may evaluate the meaning of symptoms resulting from certain foods—whether as aggravating factors of yeast-related symptoms, or whether as symptoms resulting from true food allergies unrelated to yeast.

I ask each reader to approach this as though she were the one sitting across my desk, while together we attempt to put together the pieces of a puzzle that often dates back many years. If we are fortunate, an hour and a half later we will have a strong idea of the factors that led to the problem and how we may do what is necessary to bring about its correction.

*This problem is very common in women, but just as disabling when present in men.

Yeast infects predominantly the superficial body surfaces on which it lives—skin and its continuation as the lining of the airways, vagina, and gastrointestinal tract. Such "local" infections, when not associated with symptoms elsewhere in the body, will be designated merely "superficial candidiasis."

When, in addition to symptoms at these local sites of yeast infection, "generalized"* symptoms also are arising from organs not themselves infected with yeast (as far as we know), we will refer to the condition as the "superficial candidiasis syndrome" (SCS). The relation of these ("distant") symptoms to yeast is proven when they too disappear as the local, superficial tissue infections disappear with appropriate anti-yeast treatment. The mechanism tying a distant symptom, e.g., memory loss, to a local symptom isn't known. Prime suspects would seem to be the 79 candida substances (antigens) already proven to be causing the formation by our immune systems of 79 antibodies that react in the laboratory with Candida albicans.

Before beginning, there are two points I would like to clarify. First, although I have thus far referred to "young women," this condition occurs at all ages and in both sexes; in my practice the ratio of female:male is 5:1. Naturally, symptoms of impaired hormone function may be expected to differ according to sex. Further, age will alter the way a particular symptom is described. As an example, "decreased short-term memory/concentration," described as such by an adult, will not be described by these words in a child; the likelihood is that "attention deficit disorder"—ADD—will have been invoked to explain the poor short-term memory/concentration observed in the child; presumably the same interference with brain function is simply carrying a different label.

*To avoid the possibility of confusion, we use the word "generalized" in referring to general symptoms (e.g., fever, headache, weakness) that might, for example, accompany an infection, e.g., "strep throat," "bladder infection," etc. Traditionally, such symptoms of a general nature, that often accompany a local infection, are termed "systemic." However, "systemic candidiasis" has been used to designate the highly dangerous condition of yeast infection of internal organs. (Fortunately, in recent years this form of candidiasis has been termed "deep candidiasis.") Therefore we have always used the designation "generalized" in place of "systemic" to avoid confusion with "systemic candidiasis" in referring to the symptoms distant to those at the (local) site of yeast infection.

As stated earlier but well worth repeating, the second point that deserves discussion is the attributing to "stress" of virtually all symptoms for which a cause cannot be found. This has permeated the medical profession and has for the most part superceded such terms as "hypochondriac" and "psychosomatic," but the meaning is still there. It's just that "stress" is much better accepted by the patient and by the family. After all, since "stress" in varying degree is present in everyone's life, it isn't necessary for the physician to establish this fact.

But what needs to be clearly understood is that such attributing to stress of chronic symptoms, merely because the cause cannot be found, does a great disservice to the patient, while accomplishing its goal of putting the blame on the patient and getting the doctor "off the hook"! Remember—since *everyone* has stress in their lives, there is no need to seek evidence for this "diagnosis"; it is a diagnosis of exclusion, made merely because all tests have yielded normal results.

The problem with this practice is that it assumes an infallibility in our diagnosis of conditions *not* related to stress—conditions due to "physical" (that is, non-psychological) causes. Nothing could be further from the truth!

Even more damaging to the patient is that the diagnosis of "stress" as the cause of these chronic, distressing symptoms tends to discourage further efforts to search for their true cause. In the physician's mind the diagnosis has been made—"stress" or "hypochondriasis." In the physician's mind each new symptom or episode just reaffirms the initial diagnosis, triggering yet another prescription for an antidepressant or tranquilizer.

Also published in this monograph are studies, in patients with SCS, of carbohydrate metabolism and membrane transport, both before and during treatment. The results suggest the possible mechanism of the truly pathologic craving for sugars and starches that is a major pre-treatment symptom in almost all patients with the superficial candidiasis syndrome (SCS).

<u>History of illness</u>: <u>Age at onset</u>—***"When were you last perfectly well?"*** This is a most useful way to begin because, so often, symptoms after many years have become a mixture of the

original candida (yeast) complaints complicated by side effects from drugs used in treatment.

The "chief complaint" is often the next question in the history. If you are like most patients in whom yeast has been out of control for a long time, it may be difficult for you to single out any particular symptom. Often it is loss of energy, or depression, or severe symptoms related to the menstrual cycle.

Symptoms characteristic of this condition: *Local symptoms*—We turn first to questions related to the "local" symptoms where the yeast lives—primarily skin, G.I. tract, and vagina. Symptoms related to colon function are prominent and often have been labeled "IBS" (irritable bowel syndrome). This may be manifested as constipation or diarrhea; very often patients say they alternate between the two. Even more prominent, and perhaps more distressing, are the excess gas and bloating. A young, slender woman can literally look 5-6 months pregnant from this condition. (Incidentally, this is one of the first symptoms to show marked improvement when nystatin therapy is begun.) Rectal itching is present in a fair number of patients; this too disappears quickly with the institution of nystatin therapy. Almost always colonoscopy, stool studies, and colon x-rays have been normal—often repeatedly.

The upper G.I. tract may have symptoms variously described as chronic nausea, heartburn, indigestion, and reflux. Often there is a history of oral thrush having been diagnosed and treated. Almost always the history indicates normal findings on gastroscopy and x-rays, with the frequent exception of a hiatal hernia, to which the symptoms are usually (incorrectly) attributed. With treatment, these symptoms disappear quickly, perhaps because of the proximity of the yeast infection to the fresh nystatin as it is swallowed (yet the hiatal hernia is still present!).

It is a rare woman who has not experienced the itching and discharge of yeast vaginitis. It is important to note, however, that an occasional woman does report that she has never had vaginitis, although she does have many or all of the symptoms in the gastrointestinal tract.

Finally, the skin may be the source of yeast products entering the bloodstream. "Athlete's foot," for example, may provide one portal of entry for the foreign substances (antigens) that are responsible for the 79 anti-candida antibodies that have been found in human blood.*

To summarize, the site at which the yeast invades the body's surfaces may be the G.I. tract, vagina, or skin. Each has its characteristic "local" symptoms that vary according to the point at which the yeast breaches these protective surfaces.

Generalized symptoms: We come now to the symptoms that are arising from various organs not themselves infected with yeast (as far as we know). In many ways these symptoms are the most distressing of all. They include such symptoms as lethargy, depression, insomnia (and occasionally hypersomnia), muscle and joint pain, soreness and stiffness, and ***two symptoms*** that are the most specific for this condition.

Two symptoms virtually diagnostic of SCS: The *first* is a clear loss of short-term memory and concentrating ability. This is perhaps the most distressing symptom of all to the patients; uniformly they seem more concerned with this than any of their other symptoms.

The *second* symptom is what we term "chemical intolerance." We are indebted to the late Dr. Theron Randolph for first describing this condition.

Many odors lead to distressing symptoms. Such odors vary from ordinary perfumes to pesticides, cleaning solutions, and exhaust fumes. In fact, almost anything with an odor seems capable of triggering mental confusion, weakness, even fainting. Less common but just as severe, when they occur, are reactions to chemicals in food.

In my present practice, 30% of patients are ordinary allergy patients without trouble from yeast. They do not have these two symptoms. During the years that I did internal medicine, both in

*To repeat for emphasis, these infections on the body surfaces—skin and its continuation as the mucous membranes that line two major hollow organs (vagina and G.I. tract)—are to be sharply differentiated from yeast infections of internal organs, known variously as "deep candidiasis" or "systemic candidiasis." This far less common form of infection by yeast is very difficult to diagnose and treat, is often fatal, and is mostly seen in association with conditions that severely depress the immune system (leukemia and other malignances, organ transplantation, HIV infections). It is rarely a threat otherwise.

training and in private practice, I do not recall encountering a condition that will cause these two symptoms in young patients.

Other symptoms that are very common and of great importance are those related to impairment of sex hormone function. Decreased libido occurs in both men and women, to the point of total impotence for two years in a young man previously reported (see *The Missing Diagnosis*—Chapter "Chemical Intolerance"). Probably 70-80 % of the female patients whom I see have noticed a definite loss of sexual desire and responsiveness. In women the menstrual cycle can be grossly abnormal. Periods may be skipped for many months or years, or they may occur at much closer intervals than normal. Acne is often a major problem, either adolescent or adult. Flooding, cramps, clots, and severe PMS, when added to the remaining symptoms, create a syndrome that is almost unbearable to these women.

<u>Relation to other factors</u>: A careful history should always be obtained regarding the excess use of antibiotics and steroids, or the use of birth control pills. *Very often* the reason for the breakdown in immunologic control of Candida albicans began with the use of birth control pills or antibiotics. In almost every patient the vaginitis is aggravated by antibiotics, often the diarrhea also.

An excessive intake of sugars and starches (carbohydrates) will almost always aggravate many of the symptoms. Similarly, patients who could formerly drink wine or beer with no trouble have had to leave it out of their diet because of aggravation of headache, vaginitis, diarrhea, etc. Frequently the patient will have made the observation that certain foods give trouble. Excess vinegar, for example, is a frequent troublemaker (see "Diet").

Included in this monograph is a copy of the diet that we now give to patients. This has evolved over the years, changes being made largely from patients' observations. It is less strict than that employed by some physicians. It is also less strict than I formerly used but has proven adequate in helping to reverse the loss of immunologic control of Candida albicans. Since two or more years are almost always required before there is much likelihood that treatment can be discontinued without relapse, a diet that is too strict is likely to be counterproductive. I also point out that if they eat something not recommended, any resulting symptoms will usually last no more than 3-4 days. Unless repeated too often, it doesn't seem to retard recovery.

I frequently remind patients that the diet in fact is "not so bad" in that it allows unlimited meat and fish, all vegetables, some fruit that can be peeled, and some bread as long as it is yeast free. Patients seem to miss vinegar in particular because of its presence in salad dressings, pickles, mustard, ketchup, and mayonnaise. Lemon juice provides a suitable substitute as suggested in "Diet." Also, recipes are provided for yeast-free bread, and mustard, ketchup, and mayonnaise—all made without vinegar.

Chapter 4
Therapeutic Trial

In this effort to help patients evaluate their symptoms as to whether yeast may be related to their chronic health problems, we would like to describe what is termed a "therapeutic trial." Doctors have to resort to this frequently when the results of tests are inconclusive.

For a length of time that in the doctor's judgment is reasonable, treatment is given and the effect on symptoms is observed. If significant improvement occurs, the diagnosis is probable and treatment is continued; if not, the diagnosis is ruled out and treatment discontinued. An example might be borderline low thyroid function (by blood tests). If symptoms clear (e.g., constipation, extreme cold intolerance, menstrual problems), the diagnosis of hypothyroidism is made and long-term treatment with thyroid hormone is continued; otherwise the trial of treatment yields negative results and treatment is discontinued.

Applying this to chronic yeast infections, and for about six weeks using our strict diet (see "Diet") in which both carbohydrates and yeast are limited, symptoms will often be alleviated or ameliorated, providing evidence that further treatment measures should be initiated. *Many* new patients have commented that, while awaiting their initial appointment to see me, they instituted the diet (as they understood it) and that this had helped more than anything tried in a number of years.

If the patient's doctor will prescribe enough nystatin* for about 5 or 6 weeks, this can be combined with the diet. Thus, by suppressing yeast with nystatin and diet, improvement can be so significant that it leaves little doubt as to the cause of symptoms. However, it is important to stress that, *even without nystatin*, diet alone may point strongly to yeast as the etiological agent in this long-standing, mis-diagnosed health problem. The dose of oral nystatin powder begins with 1/8 teaspoon after each meal and at bedtime, together with vaginal nystatin twice daily. It is my

*See discussion of nystatin under "Part Two: Treatment."

practice to double the oral dose each week until symptoms improve. There is no need for further increases once the G.I. symptoms have disappeared; we will have reached the dose required to kill the strain(s) of yeast harbored by this particular patient.

If the top dose of 2 teaspoons of nystatin 4 times per day, combined with diet, fails to result in significant improvement, treatment is discontinued; the "therapeutic trial" is negative. This is the top dose reported necessary to sterilize the stool and vaginal cultures for yeast.*

During such a therapeutic trial, every effort should be made to avoid antibiotics and steroids. If on birth control pills, if possible it would be wise to discontinue them for a month or two before instituting the therapeutic trial.

What we are doing with a therapeutic trial is suppressing a yeast that is in everyone, thereby suppressing as well the 30-40 foreign substances** (antigens) that are being fed into the bloodstream by Candida albicans. Some have expressed concern about killing *all* the yeast—about whether "we might need it." However, we don't need to worry about whether we need it since we can't get it out of the body. For example, yeast in the sinuses will not be reached by nystatin.

During a therapeutic trial, nystatin is also used vaginally twice daily, even in the absence of vaginal symptoms. Our goal is to suppress yeast everywhere we can reach it with nystatin. Its use is continued during the menstrual period.

---

*New England Journal of Medicine, 1981 Apr 30; 304 (18): 1057-62.

**It has been estimated that one individual has 30-40 of the 79 reported anti-Candida antibodies.

PART TWO

TREATMENT AND DISCUSSION

Chapter 5
Treatment of Superficial Candidiasis Syndrome (SCS)

Avoidance of aggravating factors: The first step in treatment is to avoid, when possible, antibiotics, "birth-control pills," steroids (cortisone, prednisone, etc.), and excess sugars, starches, and yeast in the diet.

Antifungal drugs: Nystatin is the antifungal drug that I use in bringing under control superficial yeast infections, whether acute or chronic. It is made by a microorganism that lives in the soil; it kills fungi, including yeast. Thus it too is a "product of nature," like penicillin that kills bacteria, and which is produced by the fungus "Penicillium."

This is the 55th year of worldwide use of nystatin with no reported toxicity. Rarely a patient may develop an allergic rash. Another important advantage is that yeast rarely becomes resistant to nystatin—important in that, as stated previously, 2-3 years (or more) may be needed before relapse doesn't occur on discontinuation of treatment.

Further, nystatin is poorly absorbed from the G.I. tract. This is important in that yeast lives throughout this organ. Anti-yeast drugs that are absorbed into blood on reaching the small intestine will not reach yeast living in the colon nearly so well as one that is poorly absorbed.

The main disadvantage of nystatin is its taste, but this can be disguised in various liquids. Also helpful is the old trick of not letting air out the nose until several full breaths have been exhaled through the mouth. "Hold your nose to take castor oil"—grandmother's legendary advice—was based on the fact that taste is "90% smell." Exhaling the fumes through the mouth rids the body of most of the bad taste, before resuming normal nasal exhalation.

On the following page is the information that each of my patients is given when starting nystatin.

Handout to my patients

NYSTATIN

*Nystatin is available in several forms, the powder being the most effective. 1/8 teaspoon of powder is equal to a dose of one tablet; however, unlike the tablet, when mixed and used as a liquid, the powder destroys yeast in the mouth and esophagus (bypassed by a tablet).

*Measure the powder with a standard set of measuring spoons. Do not pack the powder and do not mix the powder with liquid until just before taking.

*Keep nystatin refrigerated and tightly closed. The medicine will not spoil at room temperature, but will lose potency over time. Nystatin will degrade more rapidly if exposed to air or warm temperatures for extended periods.

Oral Administration:

* Add a few ounces of water (or other liquid) to the measured dose of powder and stir.
* Swish each mouthful for 20-30 seconds before swallowing.
* Take the nystatin orally four times per day unless otherwise instructed.
* It is important to space these doses throughout the day. Doses should be taken around breakfast, lunch, dinner, and bedtime.
* Nystatin may be taken on an empty or full stomach; however, many patients find that they are better able to tolerate the nystatin when taken with food.

Vaginal Administration:

* Obtain a box of #4 gelatin capsules from the pharmacy. Fill the capsule halfway with the same powder used for oral administration and insert vaginally.
* To fill the capsule: pull it apart and push the long end, open side down into the powder until full, then fit the halves of the capsule back together. Several vaginal capsules may be made up ahead of time as long as they are kept in a container in the refrigerator.
* Use the capsules twice per day, morning and night, unless otherwise instructed. Vaginal capsules should be continued during the menstrual period.

Beginning instructions for nystatin are as follows:

Oral Dose: 1/8 tsp. of powder four times per day.
Vaginal Dose: one capsule two times per day.

DIET IN THE TREATMENT OF CHRONIC CANDIDIASIS*

Symptoms may result when the yeast Candida albicans succeeds in penetrating tissues. Some of these symptoms result from allergic reactions to yeast products entering the bloodstream from the sites of tissue invasion, while others may be due to toxic mechanisms (non-allergic). Finally, the symptoms in the intestinal tract and vagina originate, at least in part, from the sites of tissue invasion by this fungus (mold).

Diet is important in reversing this process. There seem to be at least two ways in which the wrong foods aggravate this condition. First, yeast-containing foods may lead to an increase in symptoms that are allergically induced. Second, yeast uses carbohydrates efficiently.

There are many varieties of yeast in nature in addition to those that live on the skin and mucous membranes of animals, including humans. These yeasts are closely related biologically. Yeasts are among the normal surface organisms of most living things and are largely responsible for the decay of substances that originally were living (organic). Thus there is no such thing as a practical "mold-free diet," and any attempt to implement such a diet is futile. A diet must be chosen that is reasonable and can be followed for an extended period of time. Some physicians give a list several pages long of foods to be omitted. It is impractical for anyone to adhere to such a severe restriction of commonly eaten foods and, in my experience, is unnecessary in controlling the clinical manifestations of chronic yeast infection.

The foods that patients have learned are most troublesome should be omitted, at least in the beginning. Among others, these include fermented beverages and vinegar, and foods containing these substances. Mushrooms are fungi and should be avoided. Aged (moldy) cheeses are poorly tolerated; cottage cheese is allowed (although some physicians prohibit it also). All types of bread that contain yeast (loaf bread, rolls, crackers, pastries)

---

*Diet—Reprinted is an exact copy of our handout to patients. It includes both diet and the previous page on nystatin.

should be avoided, in contrast to cornbread or biscuits made with baking powder, both of which are allowed. Any patient who notes a particular food that repeatedly induces symptoms should, of course, add that food to the list of foods to be avoided in his or her particular case.

In identifying low-yeast foods, certain principles are helpful. Foods that can be peeled or shelled, or from which the juice can be squeezed, or that may be cut open and eaten immediately, will probably be as close to "yeast-free" as is possible. Examples might be bananas, citrus fruits, melons, peas, beans, and potatoes. However, once the inner portion of the food has been exposed to air by cutting open, peeling, or juicing, yeast begins to colonize it. Therefore foods should be eaten immediately in order to take advantage of the elimination of surface yeast. Remember also that handling the food while processing it in this way will contaminate the hands with yeast, which will, unless care is taken, be transferred to the exposed food.

A good example is the high yeast content of fruit juices that have been processed into frozen, canned, or bottled forms. For example, when oranges or apples are cut or crushed for such processing, the interval between the beginning and end of processing allows yeast to colonize the exposed fruit or juice. Contrast this to squeezing and drinking the juice immediately as a source of "yeast-free" orange juice.

There is no way to know specifically the yeast content of many foods. Labels often indicate that yeast has been added, but many times it will be present even though not indicated on the label. In general, any food that has come from a processing company is a candidate to be contaminated with yeast, either intentionally or accidentally. Also remember that preparation and cooking methods may introduce additional yeast and carbohydrates into otherwise acceptable foods. For example, meat that is barbecued has often been treated with vinegar, and that which is fried has often been breaded. It is therefore best, especially in the early stages of treatment, to eat meat and fish that have been cooked without the addition of other substances (except salt) and to rely on fresh vegetables and fruits.

The second dietary measure that can retard yeast growth in the human body is the limitation of the total carbohydrate intake. Carbohydrates, best known as sugars and starches, are present in many types of foods. In general, meat and fish are very low in both carbohydrate and yeast and are well tolerated by yeast sensitive patients, except those patients who may have trouble from *any* food on the basis of chemical sensitivity rather than carbohydrate content. (See *The Missing Diagnosis.*)

Vegetables and fruits vary widely in carbohydrate content, and this variation is largely responsible for the variation in calories for these two classes of foods. In meat and fish, on the other hand, caloric differences are due largely to fat content. A good example of the variation in calories among individual foods is that seen in the bean family. Green beans (string beans) are very low in calories, while navy beans are very high. This difference results largely from the difference in their carbohydrate content. Similarly, certain fruits are relatively low in calories and therefore carbohydrates (cantaloupe), while others are the opposite (oranges).

Restricting the total carbohydrate intake per day deprives the yeast of the principal nutrient on which it depends for maximal growth and for the formation of yeast products that may cause symptoms. With respect to yeast growth, sugar does not seem to be any more aggravating than starchy foods such as potatoes, corn, rice, and cereal grains. The carbohydrate in these foods is immediately broken into sugar molecules by the body's digestive juices so that, in effect, sugar is being eaten even though these foods do not taste sweet. (Please note this comment refers only to stimulation of yeast growth. There may be other reasons why the intake of pure sugar should be limited, primarily those related to blood sugar regulation, such as hypoglycemia and diabetes.) The fact is that pure sugar is absorbed largely in the small intestine and does not reach the large intestine where much of the yeast lives. Sugar, of course, must be counted in the total carbohydrate intake.

The degree of carbohydrate restriction must be tempered by such things as the patient's initial age, weight, growth status, stage of treatment, and other unrelated medical conditions that may require different dietary management. In the absence of other contraindications, a restriction to 60-80 or perhaps 100 grams of carbohydrate per day is well tolerated in most cases, and during the first few weeks or months of treatment adherence to the diet contributes greatly to early improvement in symptoms. The long-term management of diet in all situations must aim at a proper balance of the various classes of foods, as well as intake of vitamins and necessary minerals.

It is important to remember that restriction of carbohydrates removes calories from the diet. These must be replaced by an equal number of calories as protein or fat; otherwise the patient is, in effect, on a reducing diet and will lose weight. Most people require approximately 1800-2200 calories per day to maintain an even weight; therefore, in treating candidiasis, once excess weight has been removed, the total caloric intake must be adjusted to the point necessary to stop weight loss in that particular individual. The level of thyroid activity as well as other factors influence this. The scales are the only way of finally determining the necessary caloric intake for each individual.

To prevent further weight loss in a patient already thin, carbohydrate calories must be replaced with protein and fat calories; certain foods are helpful. Some recommended foods include meat and fish, nuts that have just been shelled, peanut butter, canned tuna packed in oil rather than water, high-calorie cottage cheese, and avocados. This is not meant to be a complete list, but indicates in general how extra calories may be obtained with a minimum increase in carbohydrate and yeast intake. Peanuts are not as yeast free as nuts with hard shells since the shell of the nut is porous and often will have a hole in it that could have provided access for yeast. Peanut butter, of course, has mold in it, but patient experience has indicated that this is not a significant problem.

Attached is a short list of foods that experience has shown to be the most troublesome. This is simply a starting point, and must be modified to individual food tolerances or allergies and according to other medical conditions in which other dietary considerations might outweigh the indication for a diet designed for yeast control. It is always wise to check with your family physician regarding any possible dietary conflict.

DIET

General Rules:

Follow the diet as strictly as possible, especially the first six to eight weeks of treatment. If in doubt about any food, do not eat it.

Limit total carbohydrate intake to 80 grams per day. Patients may want to consider purchasing a carbohydrate gram counter to assist in tracking daily carbohydrate intake. These books are available at most bookstores.

Avoid B vitamin supplements and multi-vitamins, which will contain the B vitamins. Women of child-bearing age, for whom pregnancy is a possibility, are an exception, and should be sure to take folic acid daily. All other individual vitamins and minerals, such as A, C, D, E, K, calcium, and magnesium, are allowed. Look for yeast-free brands. Herbal supplements are not allowed.

Fresher is better! In general, fresher foods will contain less mold. Keep leftovers for only about one day. Eat only freshly opened canned foods. Foods that need to be kept for an extended period should be frozen. Also, homemade sauces and dressings can be frozen in individual portions, such as in ice cube or popsicle trays.

Read Labels! Yeast is used as a flavor enhancer in many processed foods. Read the ingredients and avoid products that contain yeast or malt.

Foods to avoid:

* aged cheeses
* alcoholic beverages
* vinegar and vinegar containing foods
* soured breads and any breads or pastries containing yeast
* pickled, smoked, or processed meats or fish
* sauerkraut
* cider
* mushrooms
* anything dried (dried fruits, dried herbs, tea, etc.)
* fruit juices, unless freshly squeezed
* any other moldy or fermented foods

SUGGESTED RECIPES

Irish Soda Bread

Ingredients:

2 cups whole wheat flour
1/2 tsp. salt
1 egg, beaten
1 tbsp. honey
1 cup plain yogurt
1 tsp. baking soda
optional: 1/8 tsp. ground cardamom or 1 tsp. crushed caraway seeds or other spice of choice

Directions:

Preheat oven to 375 degrees. Stir dry ingredients together. Beat honey and yogurt into beaten egg. Gradually pour this mixture into the dry ingredients and mix together with hands. The combined mixture will be dry like yeasted bread dough. If the dough is too dry, add yogurt; if it is too wet, add flour. Knead bread for 5 minutes. Place in oiled bread pan or shape and place on oiled baking sheet. Cut two parallel slashes in the dough about 1/2 – 1" inch deep to allow dough to rise without cracking. Bake at 350 degrees for 25-30 minutes, until well browned. Bottom will sound hollow when tapped.

Yeastless Bread

Ingredients:

- 2 cups all purpose flour
- 2 tbsp. whole wheat flour
- 2 heaping tsp. baking powder
- 1 tsp. shortening
- 1/2 tsp. salt
- 1 egg, beaten
- 1 cup plain yogurt
- 2 tbsp. honey

Directions:

Preheat oven to 350 degrees. Cut shortening into dry ingredients. Mix together egg, honey, and yogurt. Add this mixture to dry ingredients and mix well. Mixture will be dry. Form into loaf or into 6 individual buns. Make a diagonal slice across the top to prevent cracking. Bake buns at 350 degrees for 20 minutes. Bake loaf at 350 degrees for 25-30 minutes.

Golden Delight Pancakes

Ingredients:

- 1 cup creamed cottage cheese
- 6 eggs
- 1/2 cup sifted flour
- 1/4 cup oil
- 1/4 cup milk
- 1/2 tsp. vanilla
- 1/4 tsp. salt

Directions:

Combine all ingredients in blender. Cover and blend at high speed for one minute, stopping to stir down once. Bake on greased griddle using 1/4 cup of batter for each pancake. Makes 20 four-inch pancakes. May be frozen.

Basic Salad Dressing

Ingredients:

1 cup low fat cottage cheese
1/4 to 1/2 cup skim or 1% milk
1 tsp. minced onion
1/4 to 1/2 tsp. seasoned salt

Directions:

Mix all ingredients in blender until smooth. Thin with additional milk if necessary. Amount of milk necessary will depend on the amount of liquid in the cottage cheese. Make dressing thicker for potato or pasta salad. Use buttermilk in place of skim milk for a tangy dressing. Store in refrigerator.

Sour Cream Dressing

Ingredients:

1/2 cup sour cream
1 tablespoon lemon juice
3/4 teaspoon salt

Directions:

Stir all ingredients together until well mixed.

Blender Mayonnaise

Ingredients:

1/4 tsp. dry mustard
1/8 tsp. salt
1/8 tsp. paprika (optional)
1/16 tsp. ground red pepper
egg substitute equivalent to one whole egg
1 tbsp. fresh lemon juice
1 cup oil

Directions:

Combine all ingredients except oil in blender. Cover and blend for 5 seconds. With blender running, slowly add oil in a thin steady stream. If necessary stop blender and scrape sides with a rubber spatula. Makes approximately one cup (sixteen 1 tbsp. servings).

Blender Mayonnaise

Ingredients:

1/4 tsp. dry mustard (heaping)
1/2 tsp. salt (heaping)
1/8 tsp. ground red pepper
2 egg whites (or egg substitute equivalent)
2 tbsp. fresh lemon juice
1 cup oil

Directions:

Combine all ingredients except oil in blender or food processor. Cover and blend until all ingredients are well mixed. With blender running, slowly add oil in a thin steady stream. If necessary, stop blender and scrape sides with a rubber spatula.

Spicy Mustard

Using half of the second mayonnaise recipe shown above, add:

1 1/2 tsp. dry mustard
1/16 tsp. ground red pepper
1/2 tsp. salt

Directions:

Blend until smooth. Refrigerate for a few hours to maximize flavor.

Homemade Ketchup

Ingredients:

10 pounds ripe tomatoes
1 large (about 1/2 lb.) onion, chopped
1 large bell pepper stemmed, seeded, chopped
1 tsp. each: celery seed, mustard seed, and whole allspice
1 cinnamon stick
3/4 cup sugar
1 cup fresh lemon juice
1 tbsp. paprika
salt

Directions:

Immerse tomatoes in boiling water for 4-5 seconds, remove from water and pull off skins. Core and quarter tomatoes into a 10 to 12 quart pan. Add onion and bell pepper. Bring to a boil over medium high heat, stirring frequently. Reduce heat and simmer uncovered until tomatoes mash readily, 20-25 minutes. Puree tomato mixture, a portion at a time, until smooth. Return mixture to pan and continue to boil gently, uncovered, until volume is reduced by half, about 1 hour and 45 minutes. Stir mixture occasionally. Put celery seed, mustard seed, allspice, and cinnamon stick on two pieces of stacked cheesecloth (6 in. square), and tie the cloth to enclose the spices. Add to pan and simmer for 20 minutes. Remove spice bag and discard. Stir in sugar, lemon juice, and paprika. Continue to simmer, stirring frequently, until ketchup is reduced to about 4 cups, about 45 minutes. Add salt to taste. Let cool and use. Ketchup can be stored in the refrigerator for up to three weeks. Freeze to store longer. Makes about 1 quart.

Immunotherapy (allergy injections): Patients will benefit from allergy injections when inhalant allergy symptoms are prominent. This is necessary to stop the sinus and respiratory infections that are leading to the use of antibiotics and steroids several times each year. In fact, often allergy-based sinus infections mark the beginning of the departure from good health in these patients. If allergy injections are indicated, referral to a competent allergist will be needed.

Duration of treatment: The long-term goal of treatment is to suppress the yeast for as long as it takes to allow recovery of the depressed state of immunity that has been demonstrated to be caused by Candida albicans. A number of studies have been published showing such immunosuppression; it has been termed "immunologic paralysis" or "immunologic tolerance."

One very important observation throws light on this aspect of treatment. It is not unusual to have a new patient totally free of symptoms after the first or second month of treatment. They then feel so well that they think they are completely cured and leave off treatment, often after the first year. Virtually every patient will relapse within several weeks. On returning to resume treatment, almost all use the same words—"I forgot how bad it was." Another 1-2 years of treatment usually is required for the immune system to have recovered to the point that it keeps the yeast from reinvading, with return of symptoms. This seems to indicate that in one year the depressed state of immunity has only partially recovered, whereas after 2–3 years of treatment, relapse often does not occur (although some patients even then require further treatment).*

---

*See "Appendix I": Long-term follow-up strongly indicates no recurrence of SCS, once it has been succesfully treated. Several cases reported in detail in *The Missing Diagnosis* were very healthy many years later, including the 2 women with long-standing illnesses diagnosed and treated as "schizophrenia."

Chapter 6
Food Allergies

As we have seen, there is one other way that patients may help with their own diagnosis. While symptoms resulting from one or more foods may be due to aggravation of the yeast problem, it is also possible that true food allergy is responsible for a particular food reaction. If undetected, one or more food allergies may cause continuation of allergy symptoms, thereby repeating the cycle of infection, antibiotics, and steroids. This could lead to the wrong conclusion in evaluating whether our therapeutic trial is positive or negative for yeast-induced chronic illness.

Of all the numerous tests for food allergies that have been devised, none have been satisfactory, presumably for one principal reason. In contrast to becoming allergic to a protein that enters the nose (grass, trees, or weed pollen, mold, etc.), proteins that enter the body through the mouth (food) have to be broken into tiny pieces called polypeptides so that they may be absorbed from the intestine into the bloodstream and used for food. Since allergy occurs to one of these tiny pieces of protein, and since the companies that make these vaccines have no way of isolating that little piece of a protein to which the patient is allergic, they send us the undigested protein to use in testing for allergic reactions. Thus we are testing for something other than the cause of symptoms.

The best way to deal with this problem is with elimination diets. Each of us can do this at home very easily. This simple procedure is based on the fact that it takes approximately 72 hours for a food to completely leave the body once we quit eating it. Therefore symptoms from food allergies normally do not improve much until toward the end of the third day; then improvement may be truly dramatic.

In searching for food allergies, it's my practice to ask the patient if there is anything he or she really likes and is eating or drinking in excess. If such a history is elicited, I find it useful to eliminate for five days* just the one or more foods being eaten in excess, merely because they are most likely to be the cause of allergies in this particular patient. Milk, eggs, and wheat are said to make up the majority of food allergies, presumably because we eat them in such excess. Also high on the list are coffee, tea, peanut butter, chocolate, and corn; but *any* food may be the offending food in a particular patient.

Beginning by eliminating a single food is fine if its intake is excessive. If the brief dietary history fails to reveal a likely candidate, other foods may be eliminated singly or in combination. If symptoms are relieved, reintroducing them individually may identify the food causing the symptoms. If confirmed when repeated, one possible food offender will have been identified.

If we are not fortunate enough to see improvement on these initial eliminations, we turn to a 5-day "strict elimination" diet. From the above statements, you can see that a *total fast* for 5 days would result in a dramatic disappearance of food symptoms. You might be allergic to many foods, but would be off all of them simultaneously.

A "strict elimination" diet is a modification of the total fast so that you don't have to be hungry for 5 days. You select one or more foods that you never or rarely eat, and that you have never eaten in excess earlier in life. This might be an exotic food, or an ordinary food that you happen not to like and therefore don't eat. We're looking for several foods to keep you from having to be hungry for 5 days; that is the only purpose of the foods to be eaten during the "strict" elimination diet. Some suggestions are fresh pineapple or coconut, any hard-shell nuts that are rarely eaten, sweet potato, and several other vegetables that most people don't eat often. In cooking these foods, only salt is used; we're not trying to see how good we can make them taste, but rather just trying to keep you from having to be hungry for 5 days.

Should you experience striking relief by the fifth day or sooner, we won't know which food or foods were responsible

*In recent years it has been reported that the elimination of milk from the body requires 3 weeks rather than just 5 days.

until we add them back. We can do this one at a time, in large quantity, adding a new food every 24-48 hours. If it appears that a certain food is the culprit, you will need to eliminate this food again for several days, then see if you can duplicate the experience. It is tedious and it is real "detective work." But it is the only really accurate way to pinpoint food allergies, at least at this time, because of the inability of the allergy supply companies to isolate the small protein fragment that is causing the trouble.

Finally, in trying to decide whether food allergies are the problem, a few very simple questions are very valuable. Do your symptoms vary with season, weather conditions, or geographic location— The word "allergy" simply means an abnormal reaction to something we are contacting. If there is a marked change in symptoms with different seasons or different weather conditions, this is not a food-type history. This indicates allergy to things in the air. These are ordinarily dust, pollen, mold, animal danders, etc.

In concluding this discussion of food allergies and how a patient may modify the diet so as to throw light on this possibility, I'd like to tell of a case I saw recently—a case that illustrates the points presented above. A 45-year-old man had been transferred to our city and had contacted the medical society for the name of an allergist to continue the allergy injections that he had been receiving for 12 years from a prominent medical school allergy department. He happened to choose me. When I asked his problem, he said, "I'm allergic to 75% of all the food I eat." Knowing that this was certainly not going to prove to be true, I asked several questions. "Do your symptoms vary with the seasons?" or "Just before or after a rain are your symptoms worse?" or "Do your symptoms go away if you travel to a different location?" The answer to each of these questions was no, "symptoms are the same every day."

In describing his problem, he phrased it this way. He said, "When I sit down to eat breakfast, no matter what I eat, within five minutes my nose starts pouring and it doesn't stop all day long until I finally can get to sleep at night." I asked what he drank for breakfast and he said coffee, as he did with lunch and dinner. I asked how much coffee he drank during the day. His answer was, "I'm a big coffee drinker." "How much?" "Twelve to fifteen cups a day."

With a history so totally negative for inhalants (things in the air) and so strongly indicating a food allergy, I told him that if he would stay off of coffee for 5 days, I was not at all sure that he needed to continue the allergy injections that he had been receiving for 12 years. He said that he would do anything to get rid of this problem. I asked him to call me at the end of 5 days.

The afternoon of the third day off of coffee he called me and said, "My nose just dried up." I asked if this had ever happened before. His answer was an emphatic "No!" I told him to continue off of coffee and call me in a week. He called a week later and said, "I've not had a single symptom." I said, "You don't need allergy shots." A few weeks later, when I received a check for the one office visit, he noted that he had had no trouble whatsoever.

This case I considered worth reporting because of the points that it illustrates. If you will get into the habit of carefully analyzing the situation *when you suddenly become worse*, you often can identify the cause. You might recall that one definition of allergy is "an abnormal reaction to something that we have contacted." This means that when we *suddenly* become worse is the best time to identify what we have just contacted.

Chapter 7
Treatment Summary

With the "therapeutic trial" for chronic yeast infections, and food elimination for food allergies, patients may be able to get a strong lead as to what is causing their chronic symptoms. At that point, except for the food elimination, in almost all cases help from a qualified allergist would be wise and would be indicated, to interrupt the repeated sinus and other respiratory infections that so often result in antibiotic and steroid therapy, which in turn repeatedly aggravate the yeast infection.

Another section in this book gives details of the diet that we use, which has proved so helpful in clearing up the chronic yeast syndrome. Some patients can get well just by identifying food allergies in the way we have outlined. This is the exact method that I use for identifying food allergies.

One final point. If the offending food is high in carbohydrate, other foods of similar carbohydrate content should also be causing the symptoms if it is yeast symptoms that are being made worse. If sugar, or other foods of carbohydrate content similar to that of the food being tested, do not aggravate symptoms, then an allergic reaction to the first food is suggested.

The same diet used for the "therapeutic trial" is the one we have found most useful for restoring immunologic control of Candida albicans. As patients improve, the diet is liberalized as tolerated. (See "Diet in the treatment of chronic candidiasis.")

Recall too, when eliminating a food from the diet, food often comes in different forms. An example is milk. Its elimination would include milk in its many forms—cheese, yogurt, ice cream. I also include butter; although it is essentially fat rather than protein; contamination with milk protein is possible. Also, "whey" and "casein" are milk derivatives often listed in "Ingredients." Read the "Ingredients"!!

Chapter 8
Autoimmune Diseases

In general terms, our immune systems defend us from factors that are a threat to our health. These include things that are foreign to our own bodies—such things as infectious agents and cells that become malignant. By "foreign" we mean those things not present in the 9 months before birth. Even transplanted organs are seen as "foreign" by our immune system and are attacked and destroyed ("rejected") unless this is prevented by drugs that deliberately weaken the immune system.

The immune system becomes a threat to health when it *mistakenly* attacks our normal tissues as though they were foreign. During the 9 months before birth, special cells of the immune system are programmed to recognize our organs and tissues and have the responsibility of preventing attacks on them by our "killer cells" that normally destroy viruses, bacteria, and other threats to health or to life itself.

It is vital, if we are to remain healthy, that these specially programmed cells, known as "suppressor cells," retain the ability to accurately differentiate between foreign factors that need to be destroyed by the "killer" mechanism, and our own normal organs and tissues that were present during the 9 months before birth. In medical terminology this is usually termed "self" and "non-self." "Self" must *not* be attacked, while "non-self" must be destroyed before it can harm us.

The importance of this normal ability of the immune system is illustrated when an organ transplant (e.g., kidney) is received from an *identical* twin. The recipient's immune system sees this organ as having been present during the 9 months before birth and "suppresses" the destructive attack ("rejection") that occurs when the donor is *not* an identical twin, in which case the transplanted kidney would be recognized as different or "foreign," and the attack would *not* be prevented by the suppressor cells. Thus it is vital to good health that the immune system always retain this ability to distinguish between "self" and "non-self." When this ability is compromised, normal tissues are attacked, leading to inflammation, symptoms, abnormal function, and possibly death.

Traditionally, the illnesses that result from such attacks on our own organs are termed "autoimmune," "auto" meaning "self." Thus "autoimmune" means an illness resulting from an immune attack on one's own tissues or organs, despite the fact that such tissue or organ was present during intrauterine life.

Once this mechanism of symptom production was discovered, each new "disease" was usually given a name that reflected the organ or tissue that was the principal target of the immune attack. On other occasions it might be named for the one who first described the illness (e.g., Crohn's disease), or given a name descriptive of a characteristic appearance (e.g. systemic lupus erythematosis, rheumatoid arthritis, etc.). Thus an ever increasing number of autoimmune "diseases" were described. There are numerous published reports of two or even three of these major "diseases" being present simultaneously in the same individual.

The current treatment of these conditions virtually always involves long-term suppression of the immune system, usually with steroids, cyclosporin, etc. Since no way has been found to suppress just the autoimmune attack, the entire immune system is weakened by this treatment. This often results in chronic yeast infections, most readily identified in women as yeast vaginitis, but often involving also the G.I. symptoms.

As we began seeing women seeking help for vaginitis, many were patients with various chronic autoimmune diseases. The first indication of a possible relation of yeast to autoimmune disease was the observation that the standard anti-yeast treatment was often associated with improvement in the autoimmune symptoms. One of the first such cases was a 30-year-old woman who reported severe chronic yeast vaginitis accompanied by severe constipation, and intermittently the diagnosis and treatment of oral thrush. These had started abruptly at age 13 years with the onset of her menstrual cycle. She had developed multiple sclerosis in her 20s. The multiple sclerosis symptoms started improving immediately with beginning yeast therapy; in 8 months she was entirely free of M.S. symptoms and remained so, including an uneventful pregnancy at age 33-34 years.*

Certainly no conclusion as to a relation of yeast to M.S. is justified in only one patient, but as the same observations were made with additional autoimmune diseases, the chance that this was more than coincidence began to look more tenable. By 1980 one or more cases representing 7 different autoimmune "diseases" led to the suggestion that these were not "diseases," but instead indicated a defect in the suppressor cell ability to differentiate accurately between "self" and "non-self," thereby allowing the killer cells to attack the patients' normal organs ("self"). It was suggested that perhaps we were dealing with "suppressor cell disease" manifested by symptoms determined by which organ (or organs) were attacked.**

Research continues into the ever-increasing number of conditions thought to result from such immunologic attack on one's own tissues or organs. There is evidence that enzymes in cell membranes are involved. The devastating effect that results on the function of many enzymes when cell membranes are more or less than normal in flexibility is reviewed in the article presented elsewhere in this book.*** Also previously published were findings of pre-treatment increased membrane rigidity in red blood cells of patients with SCS, and the rapid return to or toward normal membrane rigidity following beginning treatment of this yeast condition.****

The early improvement in Rbc membrane flexibility coincides with the early improvement in symptoms. This is illustrated in Figure 1 by the great improvement in Rbc membrane flexibility in the second patient shown. This patient's diagnosis was SLE (systemic lupus erythematosis). It was with great difficulty that

* This case reported previously in *The Missing Diagnosis* November 1985, page 88, softcover and August 1986, page 81, 2nd Edition hardcover.

** Truss, C. O.: The Role of Candida Albicans in Human Illness. Journal of Orthomolecular Psychiatry 1981; 10:228-238.

*** "Membrane Transport in Patients with Chronic Superficial Yeast Infections: Insulin Resistance, Glycosuria and the Metabolic Syndrome."

**** Truss, C. O. Metabolic abnormalities in patients with chronic candidiasis: the acetaldehyde hypothesis. J. Orthomolecular Psychiatry 1984: 13: 66-93.

her husband brought her the 2500-mile trip for her initial visit. Two months later she was so much better that she came alone to bring her son to be seen, and thus was available for repeat Rbc filtration. Her red cells that had filtered at less than 50% before treatment now filtered 100%. Again, it is important to stress that this improvement in membrane flexibility coincided with marked improvement in her symptoms of SLE.

There will always be differences among patients as to their diligence in adhering to the diet and nystatin schedule. This would have an effect on the extent and speed of improvement in Rbc flexibility. (This is illustrated in the seventh patient shown in Figure 1. This woman was a heavy consumer of alcohol, and she admittedly made no effort to decrease the quantity of alcohol consumed. After 2 months treatment, no improvement in membrane flexibility had occurred; neither had symptoms improved.)

In summary, an additional 27 years have passed since my suggestion that we are not seeing different "autoimmune diseases," but rather are seeing various manifestations of the autoimmune defect, with symptoms varying according to which tissues or organs are attacked.

The "diagnosis" should reflect this diminished ability of the immune system to distinguish "self" from "non-self." Since, as far as we know, this is a responsibility of the "suppressor cells," the name of the "disease" should reflect this fact. Until more is known about the biochemical pathways involved by which "self" is recognized and distinguished from "non-self," it seems to me that my original suggestion remains valid—that we temporarily refer to "suppressor cell disease" manifested by symptoms that reflect the organs that are attacked.

When we know more about the *normal* mechanisms involved in recognizing "self," the *abnormalities* in these mechanisms perhaps should allow a more precise understanding of the defect in suppressor cell function that is allowing the immune attack on "self." Meanwhile, the membrane abnormalities caused by Candida albicans remain a good candidate for the defect in suppressor cell function.

Two other autoimmune conditions that respond to anticandida treatment are chronic urticaria and interstitial cystitis.

Chronic urticaria: Commonly referred to as "hives," this distressing condition often goes on for many years. Some textbooks state that up to 70% of cases are "idiopathic" (cause unknown). Often the cause of hives is easily discerned, e.g., shrimp, penicillin, etc. When the cause is not apparent, the response to a brief therapeutic trial of nystatin and diet will often establish the cause as yeast; at this time there simply is no other way to make this determination. Such therapeutic trials have indicated that yeast is responsible for a high percentage of these "idiopathic" cases.

Interstitial cystitis: This very painful bladder condition, prevalent in women, is diagnosed by biopsy of the bladder lining and is considered to be an autoimmune disease. It has defied every treatment, is very painful, and persists for years. We have been able to gradually bring the pain under control by treating Candida albicans with diet, oral and vaginal nystatin, and Candida albicans extract. By using extremely dilute solutions of Candida albicans extract, temporary relief of this pain has been achieved in almost every one of the 18 patients in whom it has been tried. At first, relief is brief. Relief gradually begins to last longer; eventually an injection of Candida extract every 3–4 days is often achieved. (This technique was discussed in my second paper.*)

* Truss, C.O. Restoration of immunologic competence to Candida albicans. J Orthomolecular Psychiatry 1980; 9: 287-301.

Chapter 9
Candida Albicans and Pregnancy

The hormone changes of pregnancy lead to yeast vaginitis in approximately one-third of women. It seems logical that this would result also in an increase in the presence in the bloodstream of the 79 antigens responsible for this number of anti-candida antibodies that have been reported in human blood. (It seems probable, too, that varying degrees of yeast stimulation would be present in the remaining two-thirds of pregnant women, just not enough to seek help for symptomatic yeast vaginitis.)

Scattered reports in medical journals of babies being stillborn with extensive Candida albicans infections attest to the ability of this fungus itself to enter the pregnant uterus. Should the 79 Candida antigens also cross the placental barrier, as seems entirely likely, they too could possibly have an effect on developing organs, as well as lead to miscarriages.

Women coming for treatment of chronic yeast infections may report as many as 4 to 5 miscarriages and no live baby. Successful pregnancy often ensues once the yeast is brought under control.

In my practice birth defects are very rare in the children of women who become pregnant while under treatment for yeast. One of my regrets is that I did not have the foresight to record the number of these pregnancies, but at all times there have been several in progress. However, I always have asked about the baby. The only reported birth defect was one instance of aortic valve stenosis. Since the overall incidence of birth defects is estimated to be 4 per 100 births, the question arises as to whether suppression of yeast by treatment so reduced the exposure to yeast antigens as to eliminate one possible cause of interference with organ formation during the critical weeks of the first trimester of pregnancy.

In addition to a possible relation to birth defects, the question again arises as to whether there might be other (more subtle) impairment of various functions not recognizable as a gross birth defect. An example might be the efficiency of the immune system. In this regard, I would like to relate a case history that I found extremely exciting and suggestive of such an event.

Case Report: A 30-year-old woman came for help with a chronic problem that began with the onset of her menstrual periods at age 13 years. She developed persistent yeast vaginitis; oral thrush was diagnosed and treated on numerous occasions; and severe intractable constipation had its onset. She also had developed multiple sclerosis. With treatment of the yeast, the oral and vaginal yeast infections cleared quickly, while the constipation persisted for 2 months before it too cleared. After 8 months of treatment with oral and vaginal nystatin and diet, her neurologist reported her M.S. to be in total remission.

She remained asymptomatic for the next 3 years. At age 33 years she asked my opinion about having a baby. She said the M.S. Society cautioned against it because pregnancy was thought to aggravate M.S. (recall that pregnancy also aggravates Candida albicans).

After considerable thought and discussion with her obstetrician, it was decided to risk pregnancy with the provision that she would be on diet and nystatin from the very first day of pregnancy.

An uneventful pregnancy resulted in the delivery of a healthy baby boy with no birth defects, and a healthy mother with no recurrence of any symptom of multiple sclerosis.

The reason for presenting this case in detail is that this baby boy was 2 years of age before having his first infection—no colds, bronchitis, ear infections, etc.! In a newborn, maternal antibodies are usually gone by 3-6 months of age, at which point a baby must develop its own immunity.

Because this mother was on full nystatin (30 million units) even in the first days of pregnancy, it seems reasonable to assume that intrauterine exposure to yeast antigens would have been at a minimum for the entire duration of the pregnancy. Could this possibly account for this most unusual departure from the usual onset of infections at 3-6 months of age in newborns?

Miscarriages: At the end of the menstrual period, the uterus has shed its lining (the endometrium). Over the ensuing 28 days (approximately), with stimulation first by estrogen and then by progesterone, the endometrium again thickens and new blood vessels form; it is now ready for pregnancy.

In a normally responding woman, progesterone therapy (as in birth-control pills) will prevent menstrual periods for years. Once progesterone support is withdrawn, the uterus is unable to retain the thickened uterine lining (endometrium) and it is shed approximately 48 hours thereafter. This occurs normally when the birth-control pill is discontinued on the 26th day of the monthly hormone cycle.

In women not taking hormones, the ovary produces progesterone for approximately 12 to 14 days following ovulation; if pregnancy ensues, progesterone production continues for 9 months, first by the ovary and then by the placenta ("afterbirth"). When pregnancy fails to occur that month, the ovary abruptly ceases progesterone production. Without progesterone support, the uterus cannot retain the thickened, vascular uterine lining (endometrium) that has formed (since the last period) in response to stimulation, first by estrogen and then by progesterone. Approximately 48 hours later the uterus is again forced to shed the endometrium (the menstrual period).

"Break-through bleeding" means that a woman taking birth-control pills starts menstruating *before* the progesterone support is discontinued on the 26th day. We know the problem is *not* due to a *deficiency* of progesterone since it is being taken in pill form.

This is yet another instance of "end-organ unresponsiveness." (See Chapter 10.) It strongly suggests that "miscarriages" may occur by a similar mechanism—the uterine lining (the "end-organ") is failing to respond to the progesterone. Thus, "break-through bleeding" and a "miscarriage" are both due to "end-organ unresponsiveness," except that in the latter case there is a baby inside.

Many women who come for help with chronic yeast problems have reported multiple miscarriages as well as multiple ovarian cysts. Could ovarian cysts represent "end-organ unresponsiveness" to the normal effect of the pituitary hormones (FSH and LH) on the ovarian tissues that they stimulate? One 22-year-old woman had 6 ovarian cysts removed between ages 16 and 22 and was scheduled for a hysterectomy. After her chronic yeast symptoms were resolved, she had no more ovarian cysts. She went on to have six children!

Candida albicans and pregnancy—Summary:

1) Candida albicans is in all individuals.

2) Yeast vaginitis is stimulated in approximately 35% of pregnant women. (The yeast may well be stimulated in the remaining 65%, just not to the point of vaginitis.)

3) Seventy-nine antibodies in pooled blood react in the laboratory with Candida albicans, indicating that the foreign substances (the "antigens" that caused the human immune system to make these antibodies) came from this yeast.

4) These hypotheses are based on case reports and clinical observations; blinded studies are indicated. However, it is well to recall that "double-blind studies" rarely if ever originate new knowledge; they test new hypotheses that are suggested by observations!

Chapter 10
End-organ Unresponsiveness

Studies in 70 women with SCS included measurement of blood levels of ovarian hormones. Without exception, blood levels of both estrogen and progesterone were normal. Yet there were several indications of an impaired response in the tissues that are influenced by these 2 ovarian hormones, a condition sometimes termed "end-organ unresponsiveness." In other words, the ovaries were producing normal amounts of each hormone, despite which the tissues behaved as though there was inadequate hormone stimulation. As the yeast problem is brought under control, the response of the "end organs" returns to normal.

This problem is particularly important in women during the child-bearing years. Irregularities of the menstrual cycle may take several forms. The periods may become too close together or too far apart, or they may cease altogether for many months or even years. The following observations point strongly to impaired responses in the hormone-sensitive tissues:

a) Libido: Decreased need for sex occurs in men and women. Impotence may become a problem in men. Already reported is a young man who was totally impotent from age 28 to age 30 after the onset of SCS at age 27 years.* Eight weeks after treatment was begun with nystatin and diet, his wife became pregnant.

   Total loss of pleasure from sex is reported in an estimated 70-80% of women with SCS. The normal erotic sensation in the clitoris has been replaced by what these women describe as a "numb" or "unpleasant" feeling. There is no evidence at this time as to why this change has occurred, but fortunately the normal feeling almost always returns as the SCS is brought under control.

---

*Truss, C.O. *The Missing Diagnosis* (softcover 1985 and 2nd Edition hardcover 1986), Birmingham, AL. The Missing Diagnosis, Inc. 1985.

b) Breakthrough bleeding: Most women with SCS have tried "birth-control pills," either for contraception or in an effort to control the problems with the menstrual cycle. Many report the problem of "breakthrough bleeding," meaning simply that the menstrual period starts before "the pill" has been discontinued. Instead of the menstrual flow starting about 48 hours *after* withdrawal of estrogen and progesterone, usually on the 26th day, bleeding begins several days earlier, perhaps on the 22nd-24th day. This should not happen as long as progesterone support continues, as is true in the birth-control pill.

c) Miscarriages: Many young women report having had several miscarriages. The high progesterone levels of pregnancy should prevent uterine bleeding. Thus, as in "breakthrough bleeding," the uterine lining (the "endometrium") is not responding fully to the action of progesterone and the uterus starts to release its lining, only this time there is a baby inside!

d) "Pap Smear": Vaginal cells as seen on a vaginal slide may look as though they came from a woman with very little estrogen in her body, yet a simultaneous determination of the blood levels of estrogen are entirely normal. Vaginal cells look very different when they have responded to estrogen. Once again, the ovaries are producing normal amounts of hormones, but the appearance of the vaginal cells does not reflect this fact until the yeast has been brought under control.

e) Breast tenderness: This symptom, a normal response to estrogen therapy, is lost. This response to estrogen returns as the SCS clears; many women have reported increased breast size as hormone function returns to normal, even as body weight remains the same.

There is as yet no evidence of the mechanism responsible for diminished responses of these hormone-sensitive tissues. Once again, the previously reported increased membrane rigidity* is an

*Truss, C. O. Metabolic abnormalities in patients with chronic candidiasis: the acetaldehyde hypothesis. J. Orthomolecular Psychiatry 1984: 13: 66-93.

appealing possibility in that the sex hormones must cross first the outer cell membrane, and then the membranes of the cell nucleus, in order to act on the cell's DNA.

A frequent element in the initial history in these women is that of multiple ovarian cysts having been removed. The most extreme case was a 22-year-old woman in whom 6 ovarian cysts had been removed between the ages of 16 and 22 years. In this instance, the "end-organ" would be the ovary, while the stimulating hormones are the two hormones released by the pituitary gland in the brain—first the follicle-stimulating hormone (FSH), followed by the luteinizing hormone (LH).

These two pituitary hormones were deficient when measured in a (second) 22-year-old woman who had not menstruated for 15 months. They returned to normal when the menstrual periods resumed after 6 months of treatment of SCS. At no time were hormones administered.

It would seem to be almost a certainty that pregnancy and childbirth would be very unlikely until the superficial candidiasis syndrome is brought under control. Diminished responses in the cells of the clitoris, vagina, uterus, and breasts return to normal when the out-of-control yeast is brought under control. Particularly important are the breakthrough bleeding and frequent miscarriages; in both instances the uterus begins to release its lining even though progesterone support persists, either in the form of birth-control pills or, as found in the 70 women in whom they were measured, as produced by the ovary.

Premature births are said to be increasing in frequency. Could the same mechanism be operative as in "breakthrough bleeding" and in miscarriages? Could this be another instance of premature weakening of the ability of hormones to prevent such release? Until more is known about the mechanisms that normally prevent prematurity, answers will have to come later.

Pregnancy stimulates Candida albicans, and Candida albicans seems to interfere with "end-organ responsiveness." Therefore, suppression of yeast could theoretically help this condition if weakening of hormone suppression is important in the case of premature births.

Chapter 11
Autism

After much consideration, it was decided that my experiences with "autism" deserve a separate report. For a number of years I have been a member of the research committee of the "Allan Cott School" which became a part of Glenwood, Inc. coincident with completion of this 3 million dollar live-in facility for treatment and research into this condition.

During these years I have treated a number of children, all of whom have experienced improvement. However, other treatment methods were going on simultaneously so that it was not possible to attribute improvement to just what we were doing. One point that did seem to stand out was the occurrence of multiple ear infections.

There was one case that was treated only in my office, just with nystatin and diet. This patient's story is presented in the following detailed summary (unedited except for a name change) written by the parents. It points strongly to a relationship of autism to yeast in that improvement seemed so clearly related to the use of nystatin in this young man's treatment.

"My Brain is Clear"

"As long as he is healthy," that's what parents wish for when they are expecting the birth of a child. He was beautiful. We named him John. But John was different, very different. He was plagued by one ear infection after another. Throat and ear infections that left him screaming were treated by round after round of antibiotics. By the time he was 9 years old, he had had thirty ear infections and over 50 rounds of antibiotics. He didn't sleep at night, he pulled away from being held, and he wasn't developing "normally." Doctors assured us that he would be alright, the ear infections were delaying his speech and his actions would become normal when he got over his ear infections. He became withdrawn with repetitive and peculiar behaviors. This was not normal. His behavior turned our lives upside down. We had to find a way to reach our isolated, non-responsive, hand-flapping, compulsive acting, non-communicative son. We said, "He's in John World." A diagnosis of autism finally put a name to his odd behavior. "Autism! What's autism? What do we do? How do we get our son out of his world and in to our lives? God help us!"

God put angels in our path. The first was a friend that connected us with a behavior modification program that involved intense, long one-on-one training. John began to say words, thrive, make friends, and behave well enough to attend school. The door to "John World" began to crack open. By third grade, he was in regular classes making A's!

Then he had another ear infection. More antibiotics were prescribed. Soon after this round, John shut down. He stopped talking; his grades fell to F's. His behavior became withdrawn and regressive. Simple tasks that had been mastered were gone. After all our work were we going to lose him again?

His mother would not allow it. She contacted some of the top researchers in the country on autism to find out why this had happened and what we could do about it. She called Dr. Bernard Rimland at the Autism Research Institute in San Diego to discuss his symptoms. Dr. Rimland suggested it may be Candida Yeast. He recommended we see Dr. Orian Truss in Birmingham, Alabama, just a short drive away from us!

Dr. Truss saw John the following week and diagnosed him with chronic candidiasis. He discussed the symptoms and treatment with us, started John on a special diet that cut carbohydrates, sugars, and yeast products, and added a regime of Nystatin powder. After seven to ten days of treatment John was coming around. The fog began to lift. Within weeks we saw major improvements in his attention, health, language, and school work. We knew we were on the right track when John came in, hugged his mother, looked up and spoke his first unprompted sentence ever, "My brain is clear!"

After a year of treatment, John has never had another ear infection and has rarely been sick. We are forever grateful to the angels that have been put in our paths including Dr. Truss for saving our lost son.

Note: Although John still has autism, he has graduated from high school, attended college for a semester and made 2 A's and one B. He has an uncanny knowledge of cartoons, and daily researches new information on the computer. He has held a job at a clothing store and occasionally reminds us his brain is clear!

Mr. and Mrs. R__________, Georgia

It is well to recall that this letter was written by the parents when "John" was 9 years old and depended on their respective memories. It did not include the many details that characterize a home in which, for 9 years, an autistic child had been raised.

When on one occasion I reviewed the histories of a number of the autistic children living at Glenwood, the only thing that stood out was the large number of ear infections that had occurred and that were treated with antibiotics. Knowing (as we do) that yeast, usually Candida albicans, is in everyone and that its growth is stimulated by antibiotics, the striking improvement in this young man when treatment was begun with the anti-yeast drug nystatin seemed clearly related to suppression of this yeast. Particularly impresive was the fact, stressed by the parents, that for the first time in 9 years he spoke his first unprompted sentence, "My brain is clear." He had never in 9 years put two words together unless repeating someone's statement.

As reported in *The Missing Diagnosis,* many children who were having repeated ear infections ceased having them when nystatin was added to their treatment regimen.

In considering the possible etiological role of Candida albicans in autism, several facts are important:

1) The tremendous increase in the incidence of autism has paralleled the similar increase in the incidence

of yeast infections. As pointed out earlier, a simultaneous increase in two conditions is consistent with, although not proof of, a relationship between the two.

2) Yeast is present in everyone, based on the universal presence of anti-yeast antibodies when serum is concentrated and shown to react with yeast when the two are brought together in a test tube. This incriminates the yeast as the source of the antigens, i.e., the substances that had stimulated the anti-Candida antibodies formed by the patient's immune system.

3) Great variation in the so-called "tissue antigens" from person to person could explain why only certain individuals react with these anti-Candida antibodies, just as other diseases have been found to occur in increased quantities in patients with certain tissue antigens on the surface of their cells.

4) In the above story, John's parents reported that he had had 30 ear infections. In our first book (*The Missing Diagnosis*) a mother reported her 16 month old son was "having a new ear infection every two to four weeks, despite tubes in his ears at 10 months." This had begun after his second exposure to antibiotics. His 5-6 bowel movements per day were attributed to his being breast fed, yet the number of bowel movements immediately dropped to 1-2 per day when nystatin therapy was begun!

5) Taken together, these points certainly indicate a therapeutic trial with nystatin is worth considering. The 55 year safety record of nystatin, together with the fact that improvement occurs early, supports this as a useful test. But it must be done properly. We cannot get yeast out of the body. Therefore we are "suppressing" yeast. Nystatin *in the proper dose* kills most of the body's yeast, and diet discourages antigen production by that which we cannot kill. Remember, "John" first spoke an unprompted sentence when 9 years old, "My brain is clear."

Chapter 12
Final Thoughts

Sixty years ago the textbooks of medicine described Candida albicans as a fungus universally present as a member of the "normal flora"—a term that was meant to include microorganisms living on the body surfaces. Included were bacteria, viruses, fungi, etc. Implicit in this term was the fact that these microorganisms are present on "healthy" subjects.

Sixty years later the current textbooks say essentially the same thing about Candida albicans, with minor additions, particularly about how antibiotics, steroids, hormones, and birth control pills stimulate this yeast.

These six decades have, however, furnished the opportunity to treat many patients for chronic overgrowth of this fungus, at the same time documenting other symptoms that cleared as the yeast overgrowth was corrected. In the last 26 years, beginning in 1982, laboratory investigations added much new information regarding biochemical and physiologic disturbances associated with yeast symptoms, abnormalities that improved or disappeared as the yeast overgrowth cleared. In many instances the chronic symptoms had been given names of "diseases." This included many "autoimmune" diseases!

The following list summarizes the clinical and laboratory evidence that Candida albicans is more than an innocuous member of the "normal flora."

<u>Laboratory abnormalities</u>:

1) Membrane abnormalities—Red blood cells were unusually rigid by filtration. This abnormality of Rbc membranes was quickly corrected with anti-yeast treatment (ref. 1984 paper, fig. 5).
2) Protein—24 hour urine showed many abnormalities corrected by treatment of this yeast (ref. 1984 paper).

3) Fats—Striking abnormalities, particularly in chain length and in degree of saturation (ref. 1984 paper).

4) Carbohydrates—Impaired glucose tolerance (insulin resistance) (ref. 2009 book).

5) Acetaldehyde—A toxic product of fermentation. (These studies will be published separately.) Many additional abnormalities in blood, urine, and breath were found. The acetaldehyde studies were striking and consistent (ref. 1984 paper).

Clinical (symptoms)—Symptoms, often several decades in duration, clear quickly with nystatin and diet (ref. 1978 paper—*The Missing Diagnosis*—1992 paper).

Autoimmune—The gratifying response of a wide range of "diseases" in this category strongly suggests that yeast is interfering with the ability of the immune system to distinguish "self" from "non-self," thus allowing an immunologic attack on the patient's cells, i.e., on tissues and organs that were present during intrauterine life.

Extremely important is the finding that symptoms caused by yeast products may precede by years the "local" symptoms (vagina, G.I. tract), at which site the yeast has penetrated the mucosal surfaces. In other words, the local site from which yeast products are being fed into the bloodstream may remain symptomatically "silent" for years.

This means that an illness caused by Candida albicans may exist even though symptoms of the local site of yeast penetration may as yet be absent. Thus the distant (generalized) symptoms may exist long before there are any local symptoms to suggest candidiasis. Therefore yeast must be thought of *even* in the absence of vaginal or G.I symptoms that normally tip us off as to this etiology of the presenting symptoms.

Until a diagnostic test becomes available, a brief therapeutic trial with nystatin may be used to rule out the yeast etiology of symptoms.

Further complicating the problem is the likelihood that we encounter new strains of yeast as we go through life. DNA differences would likely ensure a different immune response to the newly acquired strain. If more difficult to control immunologically, overgrowth and symptoms might be anticipated.

An Attractive Hypothesis

Extremely elusive is "final proof." Pending that, an hypothesis to explain current observations can be very useful, in this instance helping to deal with abnormal physiology leading to symptoms ("disease"), and pointing the way to future research.

"Autoimmune disease" refers to conditions in which the immune system has, to some degree, had impairment of its ability to distinguish "self" from "non-self" so that the suppressor mechanism has begun to allow an immune attack on cells present in the uterus before birth (self). Antibodies, thus formed, react with antigens (on the cell) resulting in inflammation, impaired function, and symptoms. Often several autoantibodies will be found in the same patient, in which case the diagnosis will usually reflect the one with the most severe disturbance in physiology (and symptoms).

Suppression of Candida albicans with nystatin and diet has relieved symptoms consistently across many of these "autoimmune diseases." Yeast is universally present in humans. Further, 79 anti-candida antibodies have been found in pooled blood in healthy humans. Finally, acetaldehyde has been demonstrated in blood and breath in numerous patients with these diseases.

Patients get well or improve greatly when yeast is suppressed. Symptoms return if yeast escapes suppression by nystatin and diet—in other words, when the ability to discriminate between "self" and "non-self" regresses.

The case of autoimmune hemolytic anemia furnished objective measurable evidence of this concept (*The Missing Diagnosis*, pages 87-88). Candida albicans may just be one of a number of substances that can interfere with the protection of our normal cells and tissues. The profound stimulation of yeast by antibiotics, steroids, and "birth control pills," together with the clinical response of symptoms over a wide variety of "autoimmune diseases," when yeast is suppressed with nystatin and avoided by diet, point to this fungus as one source of one or more substances that may initiate this sequence of events. In my opinion, acetaldehyde remains a major suspect as this initiating factor (see page 147, "Metabolic Abnormalities in Patients with Chronic Candidiasis: The Acetaldehyde Hypothesis").

Proof remains elusive!

PART THREE

SCIENTIFIC
(Dr. Truss' 6th paper—not previously published.)

with contributions from:

C. Orian Truss, MD

Carroll V. Truss, PhD

Brian Cutler, PhD

Kenny Lenoir, BA

Barbara Dickey, MT (ASCP)

Lauren Graffeo, BS

Membrane Transport in Patients With Chronic Superficial Yeast Infections: Insulin Resistance and Glycosuria— The Metabolic Syndrome

(This is the first report of carbohydrate studies in women with SCS. Pre-treatment studies in 53 women were followed in 9 of them by repeated studies as treatment progressed.)

INTRODUCTION

Little is known of the effect on human physiology of the antigens responsible for the presence in human sera of 79 antibodies that react with Candida albicans, other than the immunosuppression reported by several authors.[1-9] This paper reports the results of exploratory studies seeking evidence in blood or urine of the biochemical or physiologic basis for symptoms so consistently present in patients with chronic superficial yeast* infections.

Candida albicans frequently penetrates the surfaces on which it lives — notably skin and nails, and mucous membranes of the gastrointestinal tract and vagina. Not uncommonly such superficial infections recur with increasing frequency and become progressively more difficult to treat, eventually to become intractable. Because of accessibility, yeast infections are most easily recognized and diagnosed in skin, nails, mouth, vagina, and in the diaper area. Also common, but often unrecognized, are yeast infections of the gastrointestinal mucosa, particularly of the colon and lower esophagus.

By counter-current immunoelectrophoresis, seventy-nine anti-Candida antibodies have been demonstrated in human blood, reflecting the complexity of the antigenic mixture to which the immune system has responded.[10] Several toxins add further to the number of reported yeast products, some with

* Unless otherwise specified, "yeast" refers to Candida albicans.

enzymatic activity, potentially able to affect function in one or more organs, thereby inducing symptoms.[11-12]

If one or more of these yeast products can indeed adversely affect function, it seems likely that the extent of such a disturbance would be related to the total area and depth of yeast penetration into superficial tissues and to the duration of the often repeated (or intractable) yeast infections.

Access to the bloodstream would seem to be critical, inasmuch as in healthy individuals Candida albicans is present without inducing symptoms. The duration of such access should likewise be of particular importance as it relates to cumulative effects of any physiologic abnormalities that might be induced by these yeast products.

The picture that emerges in patients with chronic yeast infections is that of a fungus that has successfully established itself in the deeper layers of superficial tissues, by virtue of which it has acquired the access to the bloodstream that is essential for chronic exposure of the body to these many yeast products. Over a period of years it may continue to spread and colonize additional sites, thereby releasing into the human bloodstream an ever-increasing quantity of these substances. Unless we are to assume no adverse effect on human health of such foreign matter entering the bloodstream chronically, it is important that a way be found to identify clinically relevant yeast penetration of superficial tissues.

Infections are typically diagnosed by cultures and by tests that search, not for the organism itself, but for past or present immunologic responses to it, e.g., skin tests and various tests for specific antibodies. A moment's reflection, however, reveals that such tests are almost always searching for evidence of contact with an organism ***not normally found*** in the human body. Since yeast is universally present, everyone having anti-Candida antibodies,[10] these tests merely tell us what we already know.

Quantitative antibody measurements have proven to be virtually useless as indicators of the extent of tissue penetration by Candida albicans. The same is true for attempts to diagnose clinically relevant yeast infections by culture.

Nowhere is the futility of reliance on cultures and serologic tests for the diagnosis of yeast infections better illustrated than in the very difficult diagnosis of "deep candidiasis,"* the highly dangerous and often fatal bloodstream dissemination of Candida albicans to internal organs, seen most often when the cells of the immune system are themselves diseased, as with HIV infections and malignancy (leukemia).[13] Daily blood cultures may remain negative up to the time of death, only to have autopsy reveal yeast infections throughout the deep organs. Equally futile have been attempts to utilize tests of the immunologic response to Candida albicans. This failure of cultures and serologic tests was stressed in the summation of a conference on this subject, leading to the concluding statement that "the diagnosis of systemic candidiasis is largely one of bedside evaluation that depends on the physician's knowledge of the manifestations of the disseminated disease."[13] Thus the diagnosis must be based on symptoms and signs — the "clinical picture"— just as in many other conditions e.g., migraine headaches, pain of any kind, depression, and virtually all psychiatric disorders.[13-17] It is unfortunate but true that for many conditions there are as yet no ways to confirm, with objective laboratory and other investigative studies, diagnoses suggested by symptoms and signs.

This, then, being the situation with this highly dangerous, deep, and frequently fatal type of yeast infection, it would seem naive to expect cultures and antibody studies to reveal clinically significant fungal penetration into superficial tissues. It has been stated that such infections of superficial tissues (also termed "chronic mucocutaneous candidiasis") may range from an asymptomatic yeast infection "under a single little fingernail," to the severe and often disfiguring infection known as "congenital mucocutaneous candidiasis."[13]

Fortunately, when superficial candidiasis has reached a certain stage, a number of symptoms of a general nature often accompanies the familiar "local" symptoms at the infected sites, thus indicating the diagnosis. Among these general symptoms are fatigue, impairment of short-term memory and concentrating

* In recent years the terms "superficial" and "deep" have often been used to designate "chronic mucocutaneous" and "systemic" candidiasis respectively.

ability, inappropriate depression, sensitivity to environmental chemicals, muscle and joint pains, insomnia, symptoms of impaired hormone function, and a truly pathologic craving for carbohydrates. The consistency from patient to patient of these general symptoms makes possible the recognition of this, the "superficial candidiasis syndrome"(SCS).** [17] The response of various symptoms to treatment (Table 1) was previously shown.[14]

It is important to point out that these symptoms are not present to any significant degree in patients presenting for treatment of ordinary allergy symptoms, in whom loss of immunologic control of Candida albicans has not occurred. Thus a patient may be extremely uncomfortable with symptoms of allergic rhinitis or asthma without incurring the fatigue, memory loss and concentrating difficulty, depression, muscle and joint symptoms, and chemical intolerance that are characteristic of SCS.

Patients for these studies were selected by careful attention to the clinical picture, including the above-described symptoms, the sequence of their onset, and their relation to the use of antibiotics, contraceptive hormones, and steroids or other forms of immunosuppressant therapy.

The difficulty of diagnosis by culture, both for deep and superficial candidiasis, is one of false negatives as well as false positives. Numerous studies have found 3%-60% positive stool cultures in healthy, asymptomatic patients, i.e., "false positives" (in the absence of symptoms).

Further, negative cultures are often found even when symptoms are relieved by anti-yeast drugs, i.e., "false negatives." Thus, if a positive culture is considered essential for the diagnosis of chronic vaginal yeast infections, treatment will be withheld in many patients chronically ill with this problem, many of whom

---

** In referring to these symptoms and to avoid confusion with the term "systemic candidiasis," "general" or "generalized" are used throughout rather than "systemic," as would be customary in denoting such symptoms as fatigue, depression, memory/concentration impairment. The presence of local mucosal symptoms accompanied by symptoms remote from the mucosal infection will be termed the "superficial candidiasis syndrome"(SCS) in this paper. When symptoms are limited to those arising at sites of mucosal penetration, i.e., local symptoms only, the descriptive designation will be "superficial candidiasis" or, alternatively, a term designating the infected site, e.g., "yeast vaginitis."

also complain of the distressing general symptoms characteristic of SCS.

This problem with false negatives was conclusively shown in a prospective, randomized, blinded study of nystatin therapy in 40 women chosen* specifically because of intractable yeast vaginitis, diagnosed repeatedly by their own physicians, and responsive (temporarily) to anti-yeast drugs.[15] Pre-treatment vaginal cultures by two techniques yielded 7 positive and 33 negative cultures for yeast; yet in all 40 women the 3 vaginal symptoms ceased on treatment with the anti-yeast drug nystatin. Therefore, despite negative vaginal cultures in these 33 women, the therapeutic response to an anti-yeast drug confirmed the yeast etiology of the vaginal symptoms, since nystatin would not resolve vaginal symptoms of the other two types of vaginitis, i.e., bacterial or Trichomonas vaginitis.

This valuable placebo-controlled study confirmed three very important points, all highly relevant regarding selection of patients for the laboratory studies reported in this paper:

1) Vaginal cultures for yeast are often negative, even when yeast is the cause of the vaginitis. If diagnosis and treatment had been based on vaginal cultures, 33 of the 40 women in this study would not have been treated.

2) Pre-treatment questionnaires confirmed that the many general symptoms previously reported[16-17] *do indeed* exist in women exhibiting symptoms and signs of chronic yeast vaginitis.

3) Finally and critically, this study demonstrated that, as treatment with nystatin cleared the 3 vaginal symptoms, 24 of the 25 non-vaginal symptoms moved in the predicted direction of improvement ($p<.0000008$).[14] The degree of improvement in four of these 25 measures reached significance ($p<.05$) despite the limited nature of the treatment.[14] (Oral nystatin was limited to 8 million units per day, whereas 30 million units per day of nystatin has been reported necessary to kill some strains of Candida albicans.[18])

* These 40 patients were chosen by and from the waiting list of C. Orian Truss, M.D.

In summary, this very important blinded, randomized, prospective study confirmed the coexistence of vaginal and general (non-vaginal) symptoms as first reported.[17] It further demonstrated that, even without immunotherapy or diet, and with only a limited amount of encapsulated nystatin administered orally and vaginally, both sets of symptoms improved significantly, thus verifying the relation of the general symptoms to the vaginal symptoms. Finally, it showed that often yeast fails to grow in cultures of the stool and vagina, even when yeast is the etiologic agent.

Membrane Transport in Patients with Superficial Yeast Infections

This paper presents results of laboratory studies in patients chosen by the same physician and who were similar in every way to the 40 women chosen for the previous blinded study.[15] Their intractable superficial yeast infections were accompanied by the same general symptoms reported earlier,[16-17] the existence of which had been verified in the pre-treatment questionnaires of the placebo-controlled study—symptoms, both local and general, that had improved with appropriate anti-yeast therapy. These laboratory studies were designed to search for biochemical or physiologic abnormalities associated with this syndrome, the symptoms of which suggest widespread, multi-system involvement.

Rationale of studies of membrane transport: By red blood cell (RBC) filtration, membranes of increased rigidity (Figure 1) had earlier been demonstrated in erythrocytes of patients with intractable mucosal yeast infections.[19] Further, in these erythrocytes the constituent fatty-acids of membrane phospholipids showed increased numbers of shorter-chain more saturated fatty acids, with a corresponding decrease in the more unsaturated fatty acids of longer-chain length.*

Membranes become more rigid with decreases in chain length or in the number of double-bonds in their phospholipid

* We are indebted to Dr. David Horribin for these laboratory studies of plasma and membrane phospholipids in erythrocytes of patients with SCS.

fatty acids. Thus, these observed abnormalities in the fatty acid make-up of constituent phospholipids of membranes were consistent with the increased membrane rigidity previously found in erythrocytes of SCS patients.

Erythrocyte membranes have been widely studied, primarily because of their accessibility. Despite the absence of a nucleus and of a citric acid cycle, erythrocytes have many similarities to other cells, including transport mechanisms such as those involved in the movement of glucose and electrolytes across the plasma (cell) membrane. Studies of erythrocytes have contributed greatly to knowledge of membrane function and, in particular, to how changes in the chemical and physical state of membranes may affect transport.

It is important to note that, in the previous studies, improvement in flexibility of erythrocyte membranes occurred as early as 8 weeks into treatment, thus coinciding with the early improvement that had occurred in both the vaginal and generalized symptoms.[19] (Figure 1)

Membrane fluidity and transport: A vast literature attests to the importance of *optimal* membrane fluidity (rigidity) for membrane transport to occur properly. (See Discussion.) It is characteristic of normal cellular function that constituent cell-membrane molecules often are in a state of constant change and motion, frequently as part of the response to a physiologic stimulus (such as insulin), or perhaps as part of an adaptation to changing environmental conditions (e.g., temperature).

Increased membrane viscosity may prevent efficient membrane transport of electrolytes, nutrients, cell products, etc., in part at least by inhibiting the conformational changes of membrane proteins and lipids often inherent in responses to stimuli, exemplified by such phenomena as the insulin-stimulated mobilization of insulin receptors from internal storage sites into cell membranes.

Because of their hydrophobic interiors, membranes allow concentration gradients to be established between adjacent aqueous compartments, without which cellular function and life would quickly cease. These lipid barriers to the movement of hydrophilic substances prevent the rapid equilibration that otherwise would occur in the concentration of water-soluble substances on opposite sides of a membrane. Mitochondria, lysosomes, peroxisomes, nuclei, other organelles, and the cell itself are dependent for their existence on such lipid barriers to the passage of aqueous solutes.

Provision must be made, however, for the controlled movement or "transport" across these lipid barriers of water-soluble substances required by, or released by, the cell or organelle. Among these are electrolytes and nutrients needed by the cell, and such products of cellular metabolism as hormones, enzymes and other proteins, and waste products, all of which must be released by the cell. Mechanisms exist for such controlled movement across membranes.

In SCS patients, the demonstrated increased rigidity of erythrocyte membranes implies a similar abnormality of cell membranes throughout the body. (See Discussion.) Thus the potential exists for abnormal membrane transport to occur in any organ, furnishing one possible mechanism for the multi-system nature of symptoms exhibited by patients with SCS.

Membrane transport studies in patients with SCS: In vitro study of human cell membranes is difficult except for erythrocytes and other cells accessible in peripheral blood. An indirect approach that *is* feasible in humans, and that was chosen for this study, is to evaluate one or more *functions* of a membrane in lieu of studying the membrane itself. Numerous studies have demonstrated, both in vitro and in vivo, that manipulation of membrane fluidity affects many transport and enzymatic functions, including the physiologic response that normally follows the binding of insulin to its membrane-bound receptor. (See Discussion.) Such studies strongly indicate the importance of *optimal* membrane fluidity in the physiologic responses to insulin.

Because of these previously demonstrated abnormalities in erythrocyte membranes of patients with SCS, studies of membrane transport were initiated in 53 women. Post-treatment studies in 9 of these 53 patients allowed evaluation of 1) the effect of therapy on pre-treatment biochemical and physiologic abnormalities, 2) how the latter are correlated with symptoms, and 3) the relative contribution of diet, nystatin, and immunotherapy to the resolution both of chronic symptoms and of pre-treatment laboratory abnormalities.

As stated in previous studies, the striking improvement in erythrocyte flexibility occurred early in treatment, thus coinciding with the early improvement in the symptoms of SCS (Figure 1).[19] This implies early improvement in membrane function (transport), if indeed increased rigidity and abnormal transport had been responsible for the pre-treatment symptoms and laboratory abnormalities.

Pre-treatment data were compared to data of controls as well as to established normals when available. Repeat studies over time in this subset of patients (n=9) allowed evaluation of the effect of treatment on blood and urine abnormalities found in the pre-treatment studies. Two approaches were chosen: 1) transport from and into the bloodstream, and 2) transport from the lumen of the nephron.

Transport from and into the bloodstream: Transport of glucose and free fatty acids (FFA) between bloodstream and cells was evaluated by the oral 2-hour glucose tolerance test (GTT). In this way membrane transport of glucose could be monitored as it moved *from* extracellular (plasma) to intra-cellular sites, primarily across cell membranes of skeletal muscle. At the same time, the movement of free fatty acids (FFA) *into* the bloodstream was measured at the same intervals.

The 2-hour GTT was attractive for several reasons. First, normals are well-established because of its use in the diagnosis of diabetes mellitus. Second, it provided a means of evaluating the handling of carbohydrates in patients who exhibit a consistent, pathologic craving for sugars and starches—that is, a pathologic craving for glucose molecules. Third, since most of the glucose leaving plasma enters skeletal muscle, it provided a means of estimating transport of glucose across the membranes of skeletal muscle cells. This is particularly important in view of defective transport into skeletal muscle cells that may occur in patients with NIDDM (non-insulin-dependent diabetes mellitus).

Plasma insulin was measured each time glucose was determined. This allowed an estimate of insulin sensitivity. In response to a standard glucose load, the amount of insulin released by the pancreas suggests the degree of insulin sensitivity. The degree of reduction in insulin sensitivity ("insulin resistance") is estimated by the amount of insulin needed to affect the transport of glucose. When insulin resistance is mild, the extra insulin released by the pancreas maintains a normal GTT; this is termed "hyperinsulism." As the insulin resistance increases in severity, even high blood insulin levels are not adequate to maintain normal glucose transport. The GTT is then said to be "impaired." Eventually, the loss of sensitivity to the actions of insulin may become so extreme that the fasting and/or 2-hour blood glucose is elevated to the degree required for the diagnosis of NIDDM. (See Discussion.)

Other substances in blood that may be abnormal when resistance to insulin extends to other functions of this hormone were also measured. These included human growth hormone (HGH), dehydroepiondrosterome sulphate (DHEA-S), C-Peptide, total testosterone, free testosterone, free testosterone percentage of total, and sex hormone binding globulin (SHBG).

Transport from the lumen of the nephron: Glomerular filtrate as it enters the nephron is essentially plasma without blood cells and serum proteins. Thus, the concentrations in Bowman's capsule of glucose, electrolytes, and other substances will approximate that of plasma. Yet glucose and other solutes may be totally absent, or present in much reduced quantities, in the fluid leaving the nephron. Possibly nowhere in the body are transmembrane pumps as busy as in the nephron, conserving needed constituents of the glomerular filtrate while allowing unneeded substances to pass, or even actively secreting (across membranes) other (waste) products not present in the glomerular filtrate.

Membrane transport in the proximal tubule begins with the transport of glucose and other solutes from glomerular filtrate into the cells that line the lumen of the nephron, i.e., across the cell's "luminal" membrane. Transport continues from within the cell, across its basolateral membrane into extra-cellular fluid, and ultimately into the blood leaving the kidney. Defective membrane transport, across either the luminal or basolateral membranes of the cells that line the nephron, leads to abnormal conservation of substances normally extracted from glomerular filtrate as it passes through the nephron. This results in increased concentrations of these substances in the now-modified glomerular filtrate that emerges from the distal end of the nephron (urine).

To assess transport across membranes of the cells of the nephron, blood and urine specimens were obtained at fasting and at each 30-minute interval of the 120-minute GTT, great care being taken to ensure that the bladder was emptied completely each time. Because the glucose concentration of glomerular filtrate is essentially that of plasma, each determination of plasma glucose also represented the glucose level in glomerular filtrate entering the nephron at that moment. Also, it should be noted that the plasma glucose level at each 30-minute time point represented the glucose concentration of fluid entering the nephron, both as the ending level for the previous 30-minute interval and the beginning level for the upcoming interval.

Because each interval began with an empty bladder, urine collected 30-minutes later represents glomerular filtrate that has been modified by membrane transport during that particular 30-minute interval, as it passes through the nephron. Measurement of glucose in the urine therefore estimates the efficiency of membrane transport (conservation) of glucose during the previous 30-minute interval. The concentration of glucose entering the nephron will range between the beginning and ending *blood* glucose level for a given 30-minute interval.

Twenty-four hour urine specimens were collected prior to the GTT, to allow measurement of various substances normally conserved by the kidney (phosphorus, magnesium, etc.), in the hopes that this would provide an estimate of total body stores that perhaps are affected by long-term wasting of substances normally reabsorbed from glomerular filtrate.

All data were compared to controls as well as to established normals when available. Post-treatment studies (one or more) were obtained in 9 women on full treatment, and in 4 patients on partial treatment. Statistical analyses were by student's T-test. These studies revealed the following:

Pre-treatment:

1) Impairment of transport of glucose from the bloodstream into cells in response to insulin ("insulin resistance"),

despite serum insulin levels elevated as much as ten times those of controls;

2) Impairment of insulin-driven transport (conservation) of glucose into and out of nephron cells, resulting in glycosuria even when the glucose load was light, i.e., at very low blood sugar levels;

Normally the two kidneys combined can conserve virtually all glucose filtered until the blood glucose reaches 180-200 mg. In these SCS patients glucose wasting in the urine occurred, in many instances when the blood sugar was as low as 60-80 mg. Glycosuria at these very low blood sugar levels indicates marked impairment of glucose transport across the membranes of the cells of the nephron, much glucose never leaving the glomerular filtrate during its transport through the nephron.

3) Impairment of insulin inhibition of FFA release from adipose cells, resulting in elevation of FFA levels in the blood;

Post-treatment:

1) Striking improvement in membrane transport of glucose, in insulin sensitivity, and in plasma FFA levels with treatment that resolved long-standing symptoms associated with superficial yeast infections;

2) Finally, by grouping patients according to treatment protocol, an estimate was possible of the relative contributions of the 3 components of treatment in the alleviation of symptoms and correction of the defective transport present prior to treatment.

The treatment protocol included oral and vaginal nystatin, low carbohydrate-low yeast diet, and immunotherapy.

MATERIALS AND METHODS

Prior to beginning a 120-minute glucose tolerance test (GTT), blood and urine were collected after a 12-15 hour fast. Each subject was then given 100 grams of glucose orally. Blood and urine specimens were obtained at 30-minute intervals for 120 minutes, the bladder being emptied completely each time.

Each subject was given 7 ounces of water three times during the first 90 minutes of the test to assure adequate urine flow.

Each 30-minute urine sample was measured and tested for glucose with a Combistick 10 (Boehringer-Manneheim) and by the glucose oxidase method. Urines were then frozen at –85°C for further testing.

Blood was centrifuged, separated, and the serum tested for glucose by the glucose oxidase method according to the Keston method[20] modified by Trendor.[21] After removal of a sample for determination of free fatty acids (FFA), serum samples were frozen at –85°C for subsequent testing.

Serum samples were analyzed for insulin by solid-phase radioimmunoassay. Additional tests at time 0-minutes included the following: Human growth hormone (HGH), dehydroepiandrosterone sulphate (DHEA-S), C-peptide, free and total testosterone, and sex hormone binding globulin (SHBG), all measured at Alabama Reference Laboratory using standard methods.

Analysis for non-esterified fatty acids utilized the Test Kit from Wako Chemicals. Briefly, non-esterified fatty acids in serum form acyl-CoA when treated with acyl-CoA synthetase in the presence of ATP, magnesium cations, and CoA. Acyl-CoA is then oxidized by acyl-CoA oxidase to produce H_2O_2 which, in the presence of added peroxidase, results in the oxidative condensation of 3-methyl-N-ethyl-N (B-hydroxy-ethyl) analine with 4 amino-antipyrine to form a purple colored adduct. The amount of FFA in the sample is then determined from the OD measured at 550μIU.

Each patient was instructed to bring a 24-hour urine specimen ending on the morning of the GTT. These specimens were measured and tested for glucose with a Combistick 10 as well as by the glucose oxidase method. For later testing, specimens were then allocated to different tubes and frozen at –85°C. Subsequent analyses included creatinine, sodium, potassium, uric acid, magnesium, calcium, and phosphorus.

Subjects: The pre-treatment GTT data are for 53 women (Table 2A). As treatment progressed, all studies were repeated one or more times in a 9-patient subset of these subjects. The data for these 9 patients, receiving full treatment and with no missing data, are presented.

Additionally, similar studies were carried out in 13 women who had already undergone long-term treatment. The purpose of this was to evaluate the effect of such long-term treatment in a small number of subjects in every way comparable to those in this study, except that they lacked pre-treatment studies.

Thus there were 66 women in four groups designated A, B, C, D, with five additional women serving as controls. Groups B and C are composed of the same 9 patients, thus providing pre- and post-treatment "within-subject" comparisons (i.e., each subject served as her own control). The matched controls were 5 women who presented no illness, and no symptoms or signs of chronic yeast problems; these comprised Group E.

Table 3

Female Groups

Group A	n=44	Pretreatment only
Group B	n=9	Pretreatment testing identical to Group A except these 9 patients were restudied during treatment. (For some statistical comparisons, these subjects were pooled with the 44 subjects in Group A.)
Group C	n=9	Post-treatment data of patients in Group B, obtained at various times during treatment
Group D	n=13	Post-treatment data (only) of patients who had already received long-term treatment.
Group E	n=5	Controls

Substances assessed during GTT: Venous blood samples were taken at 0, 30, 60, 90, and 120 minutes from the 4 SCS groups and from the control group. At each of the five sampling times during the GTT, measurements were obtained for blood levels of glucose, insulin, and free fatty acid (FFA). Further, urine glucose was determined at each interval.

Other substances that have been reported to be influenced by insulin were analyzed in the time 0-minutes. Data on the following substances were determined: HGH, DHEA-S, total and free testosterone, SHBG, weight, height, waist and hip circumference, body mass index, and systolic and diastolic blood pressure. (These will be reported separately.)

Data Analysis

Data for glucose, insulin, and FFA were analyzed in four ways: 1) average of the 5 sample means; 2) areas under the GTT curve (AUC); 3) peak of sample means (n=9) at each sampling time during the GTT; and 4) concentrations at 120 minutes.

Average of the sample means. The means of glucose, insulin, and FFA at each of the five sampling times of the GTT were computed and averaged for each group (A, B, C, D, E). Figure 9 plots the data of the 4 patient groups (A, B, C, D).

Area under the GTT insulin and FFA curves. The total of the response of each substance measured is computed as a straight-line approximation to area under the GTT curve.*

Analyses by peak concentration of glucose, insulin, and FFA. This is for 9 patients with full treatment (Figure 10). The mean change pre to post in peak levels was computed for each of the 9 patients, and the mean change in peak calculated for each sampling time. Mean change in peak was tested for significance.

Concentration at 120 minutes of glucose, insulin, and FFA. The change in average concentration at 120 minutes for the 9 patients was the plotted variable.

---

* Explanation of the straight-line approximation method. (This method does not take into account slight variations due to using straight lines from one sampling time to the next.) The area under the curve of sample concentrations at each sampling time, using the mid point between each GTT sampling time, is computed treating each of the four 30 minute GTT sampling intervals as having a width of 1 and a height equal to that of the mid point between each sampling time.

RESULTS

Insulin resistance of progressive severity (Figure 2) was the most striking abnormality in these patients, including one whose 120-minute blood glucose by GTT was 201 mg%, thus meeting the criterion for the diagnosis of type II diabetes mellitus. Twenty-one months of treatment returned her insulin sensitivity to normal; however, regression in insulin resistance was seen after six months without treatment (Figure 3A–3H). A second patient, almost diabetic before treatment with a 120-minute blood glucose of 194 mg%, showed marked improvement after one year of yeast treatment (Figure 8).

Additionally, glucose conservation was defective. Glucose passing through the nephron appeared in the urine at blood sugars as low as 65-70 mg% (Figure 6A). Post-treatment results showed disappearance or clear improvement of urine glucose levels in all patients who exhibited pre-treatment glycosuria (Figure 6B).

Finally, elevated plasma free fatty acids (FFA) were found in a majority of these women, indicating resistance also to insulin's role in preventing the release of FFA from triacylglycerol stores (Figure 4D). Five out of nine patients showed elevated FFA before treatment, all of which became normal with treatment (Figure 4E).

Fifty-three women were studied prior to beginning treatment. These pre-treatment data are presented in Section I below; they include studies of both urine and blood. Section II includes post-treatment studies in 9 of these 53 women, with comparisons to their pre-treatment findings.

Also studied were 13 asymptomatic women who had been treated for a number of years (who therefore had no pre-treatment data), but in whom the presenting symptoms were identical to those of the 53 women in the present study. It was felt that findings in these 13 women should give an idea of what might be expected after a comparable period of treatment in the 53 women studied prior to treatment. Results thus are presented as follows:

I. Pre-treatment studies in 53 women:

1. Glucose tolerance studies, including blood levels of glucose, insulin, and FFA at each interval of the GTT (Table 2A)
2. Studies of glucose reabsorption in the nephron (Figure 6A, 6B)
3. Electrolyte excretion in 24-hour urine collections (Figure 7A, 7B, 7C, 7D)
4. Additional data for parameters known to be influenced by insulin (to be presented at later)

II. Post-treatment studies:

1. Repeat in 9 of the 53 women of the same tests obtained pre-treatment (Figure 4A, 4B, 4C, 4D, 4E, Figure 6B, Figure 9, Figure 10)
2. Same studies as in section above in the 13 women already treated for several years, and whose initial complaints were in every way comparable to those of the present subjects (Figure 9)

Table 2A provides the data for Groups A, B, C, and D. The number of data for each point is shown in all tables, since instances of missing data points were frequent, primarily because venipuncture often was difficult. Also provided in Table 2 are 1) significance of differences between pre-treatment means of Groups A and B, showing that the nine patients in Group B are a true subset of the fifty-three patients in Group A; and 2) pre/post change scores and their significance for the nine "repeated measures" patients (Group B vs. Group C).

DISCUSSION

Defective membrane transport as demonstrated in these studies provides a plausible explanation for what has been one of the most perplexing aspects of the superficial candidiasis syndrome—that symptoms referable to so many systems of the body are consistently present in women subject to intractable or frequently recurring vaginal yeast infections.

Because of feasibility, these studies focused primarily on the transport of glucose from the bloodstream and from glomerular filtrate, and on the transport of FFA into the bloodstream from adipose cells. However, similar impairment of transport of other substances might well be present—even expected—since for many substances defective transport has been shown when membranes are abnormally rigid as had been found in earlier studies in patients with SCS.[19]

Further, resistance to other actions of insulin was suggested in these patients by abnormalities in sex-hormone binding globulin, DHEA-S, and free testosterone.* In view of insulin's many regulatory roles, findings suggestive of impaired responses to insulin (glucose transport from blood and proximal renal tubule, FFA into blood) suggest, as potential causes of the chronic symptoms, similar defects in transport in other organs, with consequent abnormalities in additional physiologic processes subject to regulation by this hormone.

Recognition of yeast as the cause of these multi-system complaints has been made more difficult in that abnormalities are rarely found following appropriate investigation of individual symptoms. Almost inevitably this leads to symptoms being attributed to "stress," and to the recommendation of psychiatric consultation.

It is highly relevant, however, that patients from widely diverse areas describe the very same symptoms. This was true even before the first publication describing this syndrome.[17] It is inconceivable, if these symptoms were indeed based on

* To be reported separately.

psychoneurosis, that individuals from different areas of the United States, as well as from other countries, and with no prior knowledge of this concept, would consistently describe the identical symptoms characteristic of this condition—fatigue, depression, decreased short-term memory and concentrating ability, chemical intolerance, muscle and joint pains, and a craving for carbohydrates in their diet. It is important to note that this partial list of SCS symptoms is not described by patients who present for treatment just of allergies (such as rhinitis and asthma), but are unique to those patients presenting with chronic superficial yeast infections of the vagina and/or GI tract, almost all of whom also have respiratory allergies.

As stated earlier, in the placebo-controlled, randomized study of nystatin therapy in 40 women chosen specifically because of intractable yeast vaginitis, pre-treatment questionnaires easily confirmed the existence of these multi-system complaints.[15,22] The question then to be answered was whether these severe and chronic "general" symptoms were indeed of psychosomatic origin, or whether chronic exposure to the many toxins and antigens of Candida albicans, reaching the bloodstream from the "local" mucosal yeast infections of the vagina and/or GI tract, was inducing symptomatic biochemical and physiologic abnormalities not revealed by the usual investigative procedures used in clinical medicine.

In this controlled study of nystatin vs. placebo in women with chronic, intractable yeast vaginitis, improvement or disappearance in 24 of the 25 general symptoms ($p<.0000008$)[14] accompanied disappearance of the 3 vaginal symptoms. Relief of the many general symptoms—coinciding as it did with relief of the vaginal symptoms, and coupled as it was with clearing of the pre-treatment biochemical abnormalities found in this study—leaves little doubt as to the etiologic role of Candida albicans in this syndrome (SCS).

Overall Picture: The results of these studies point to insulin resistance and impaired membrane transport of glucose, both from the bloodstream and from the glomerular filtrate (conservation), despite greatly increased amounts of insulin released by the pancreas following glucose ingestion. Such failure of normal responses to insulin was further manifested as loss of insulin suppression of FFA release from adipose cells, resulting in increased FFA in the bloodstream. Finally, the possibility that impaired reabsorption in the nephron may have led to total body electrolyte deficits was suggested by very low levels of phosphorous, magnesium, and calcium in pre-treatment 24-hour urine measurements.

Transport of Glucose from Blood—Pre-Treatment: In these young women the pattern was that of impaired sensitivity of the insulin-stimulated transport of glucose from blood into cells (primarily skeletal muscle). The degree of this loss in insulin sensitivity varied from mild to severe (Figure 2)—from a greater than normal insulin response adequate to maintain normal glucose tolerance (hyperinsulinism) to an insulin response unable to prevent an impaired GTT, in one instance reaching ten times that of controls (Figure 3A). In this 36-year old woman the 120-minute glucose remained at 201 mg% despite a 120-minute blood insulin level of 610mIU/mL (Figure 3B)—10 times that of controls. Thus, in this patient insulin resistance had reached the degree of severity that justified the diagnosis of non-insulin dependent diabetes mellitus (NIDDM). This patient's history and response to treatment are presented in detail elsewhere as "Case One."

The range in resistance from mild to severe in these women is similar to that seen as insulin resistance progresses over many years in a diabetic's sibling who too eventually becomes diabetic. Diabetic-prone monkeys demonstrated similar progression in insulin resistance when followed for 17 years.[23-24]

Transport of Glucose from Blood—Post-Treatment: Repeat studies in a subset of these patients showed that, as treatment resolved mucosal yeast infections and their associated local and general symptoms, insulin resistance decreased in severity or resolved completely as manifested in fasting, peak, and 2-hour insulin levels (Figure 4A, 4B, 4C). In these women, each of whom was treated with diet, immunotherapy, and oral and vaginal nystatin, repeat oral GTTs showed striking improvement in glucose tolerance; and this was brought about by much less insulin. This increase in insulin sensitivity accompanied clearing of the local and general symptoms of SCS.

Two other women who stipulated their unwillingness to adhere to the diet showed moderate improvement in symptoms with little change in insulin sensitivity as measured by GTT (Figure 5A, 5B), in contrast to the greater improvement in insulin sensitivity (Figure 5C, 5D) and symptoms seen in still two other women treated just with nystatin and diet, who did not receive immunotherapy because, in addition to SCS, multiple sclerosis was present.

Thus, in these four subjects nystatin and diet alone yielded better results than nystatin and immunotherapy alone, while maximum improvement in both symptoms and insulin sensitivity was achieved in the 9 subjects receiving full treatment with nystatin, diet, and immunotherapy.

Transport of Glucose in the Nephron—Pre-Treatment: In addition to the impaired membrane transport of glucose from the bloodstream, strong evidence was found of impairment of the normal insulin-stimulated movement of glucose and other solutes across the membranes of the nephron, primarily in its "proximal convoluted tubule" (PCT) segment.

One important role of insulin is to facilitate reabsorption in the nephron (membrane transport) of certain substances to be conserved. These include glucose and certain amino acids and electrolytes. The luminal membranes of the cells of the proximal tubule are rich in insulin receptors; normally only a small amount of glucose is able to escape in the urine.

Conservation of solutes by the kidney involves transport, first across the luminal and then across the basolateral membranes of the cells of the nephron. Such transport conserves virtually all glucose filtered by the glomerulus, the normal 24-hour urine output being approximately 125 mg. The finding in this study of large amounts of glucose in the pre-treatment 24-hour urine is in itself abnormal.

Powerful evidence of impaired membrane transport of glucose in the nephron was revealed when, at fasting and at each 30-minute interval of the GTT, urine glucose levels were correlated with blood glucose levels and hence with the glucose concentration in the glomerular filtrate entering the PCT. By having patients empty the bladder *completely* each time, glucose emerging in the urine during a particular 30-minute interval would have done so as the blood sugar ranged from its beginning to its ending concentration for that particular 30-minute interval. (By way of illustration, if blood sugars were 115 mg% at 90 minutes and 80 mg% at 120 minutes, glucose present in the 120-minute urine specimen would have passed through the nephron while the blood sugar, and therefore the concentration of glucose entering the nephron, was ranging between 115 and 80 mg%.)

Forty-four patients were studied in this manner. In 35 of these 44 patients glucose was present in the urine at blood sugar levels far below those at which glycosuria should occur (Figure 6A). There should be no sugar in the urine at blood sugar levels such as these, since the estimated 2 million nephrons in the two kidneys have the ability to conserve essentially all glucose entering the nephrons until the total glucose load exceeds their combined capacity; this is reached at blood sugar levels of 180-200 mg%.

Transport of Glucose in the Nephron—Post-Treatment: Of the 9 patients studied with repeat GTTs, 5 had significant glycosuria prior to treatment. In 4 of these 5 patients glucose was absent from the urine after treatment, and was greatly reduced in the 5th patient (Figure 6B).

The pre-treatment results indicate defective membrane transport of glucose across the membranes of cells of the nephron, primarily in its proximal segment. Since insulin facilitates this process, insulin resistance in the nephron is a plausible explanation of the striking impairment of membrane transport of glucose in the nephron. This concept is strengthened in that the improvement in glucose conservation in the nephron coincided with improvement elsewhere in the body in insulin sensitivity for glucose and FFA.

Transport of Electrolytes in the Nephron Pre- and Post-Treatment: The finding of gross deficits in the 24-hour urine content of certain electrolytes and other constituents further suggests defective transport (Figure 7A, 7B, 7C). Among the actions of insulin is facilitation of transport in the nephron of certain ions, particularly sodium and phosphorous, which move in concert with glucose as they too are conserved in the nephron. With excessive loss of electrolytes over time as a result of defective membrane transport, a total body deficit might well develop. This is suggested by the very low 24-hour excretion of (particularly) phosphorous and magnesium.

As may be seen in "Case One," with treatment definite change toward normal occurred in the excretion of magnesium, phosphorus, and calcium, each of which had been low prior to treatment (Figure 7D). It is not possible to know the extent to which insulin resistance is responsible for these consistent and severe electrolyte abnormalities, but they suggest long-standing defects in conservation of electrolytes in the nephron.

Transport of FFA into the Bloodstream—Pre- and Post-Treatment: Further evidence of insulin resistance was found in the elevated bloodstream levels of FFA, the release of which from adipose cells is strongly inhibited by low levels (20mIU) of insulin (Figure 4D). The strong move to or toward normal with treatment (Figure 4E) indicates restoration of insulin inhibition of lipoprotein lipase and therefore of FFA release. The elevated blood levels of FFA also suggest the use of FFA rather than glucose as the primary cellular fuel. (See Glucose-Fatty Acid Cycle.)

Summary: These studies indicate 1) impaired membrane transport of glucose from blood across membranes of (primarily) skeletal muscle cells, 2) defective membrane transport of glucose and electrolytes in the nephron, and 3) loss of inhibition of the release of FFA from adipose cells into the bloodstream. Since insulin action is critical to each of these processes, these findings suggest that insulin resistance may be present in each instance. This insulin resistance clears with treatment that clears the local and generalized symptoms of chronic mucosal yeast infections and, as previously shown (Figure 1), restores flexibility to cell membranes.

These findings further suggest the possibility of widespread functional abnormalities in membrane transport, potentially capable of affecting biochemical and physiologic processes in cells and organs throughout the body. A clinical syndrome encompassing symptoms referable to multiple organs becomes plausible.

Membrane Rigidity and Transport

Membrane Rigidity: As noted earlier, numerous studies have demonstrated impairment of transport when membranes become more rigid, and increased rigidity of erythrocyte membranes had earlier been reported in patients similar in every way to patients in this study[19] (Figure 1).

If erythrocyte membrane rigidity is representative of that of membranes in general, and if the increase in membrane rigidity is sufficiently severe as to impair transport into and out of cells, then multi-system symptoms would be consistent with the resulting impairment of physiologic processes in the various organs.

Indeed, the status of erythrocyte membrane flexibility has been found to correlate with that of membranes in the liver and other organs. Further, in certain congenital conditions characterized by enzyme defects that result in increased membrane rigidity, such rigidity has proved to be a general phenomenon. Also, since membrane phospholipids of the various organs are synthesized in much the same way, it seems likely that the demonstrated abnormalities in membrane phospholipids would not be unique to erythrocyte membranes. Finally, plasma phospholipids in these patients showed the same pattern of fatty acid abnormalities found in erythrocyte membranes;[19] this would tend to affect membranes throughout the body, since membrane phospholipids adopt the pattern of the phospholipids of the plasma in which they are bathed.

Membrane Fluidity and Function: In view of the increased membrane rigidity present in patients with SCS,[19] it is relevant to consider how the functions of a membrane are affected by its state of fluidity. Also of interest, in view of the findings in the patients in this study, is a brief consideration of the interrelationship of glucose and fatty acid metabolism, the influence of insulin on each, and the "glucose-fatty acid cycle" as proposed by Randle.[25]

Changes in membrane fluidity may be pathologic but also may be physiologic, as in an adaptation to an environmental factor such as temperature. Pertinent to abnormalities found in these patients are examples from the literature illustrating the effect of increased membrane rigidity on membrane function.

Among these are functional impairment of membrane-bound enzymes,[26-30] of amino acid transport,[31-32] and of glucose transport.[33] Among specific membrane functions that have been shown to be affected adversely as membranes become more rigid are facilitated diffusion,[34] Na^+-K^+ ATPase function,[35-38] mitochondrial enzyme function,[39] and the function of the Ca^{2+} ATPase pump in the sarcoplasmic reticulum.[40] Many of the factors that influence membrane rigidity have been reported in patients with NIDDM;[41-43] this is relevant since NIDDM represents insulin resistance that is severe ("Case One"). Reviews of this vast literature are available.[44-47]

It does not necessarily follow that the abnormal movement of glucose, FFA, and electrolytes in these patients is due entirely to the rigid membranes. What is clear, however, is that many symptoms were present at the time that these membrane and transport abnormalities were present but were absent following treatment that returned to or toward normal the flexibility of the erythrocyte membranes.[19]

Overview of Pre-Post Treatment Studies

Post-Treatment GTT and FFA: As treatment resolved the mucosal yeast infections and the associated local and general symptoms, glucose tolerance improved or became normal even as blood insulin decreased, both fasting (Figure 4A) and peak (Figure 4B), often to levels no higher than those in control patients. Concomitantly, blood levels of FFA decreased sharply, in most cases into the normal range (Figure 4E). Thus, with the return to normal of glucose transport from the bloodstream came the return of inhibition by insulin of free fatty acid transport from adipose cells into the bloodstream. Glucose then moved normally across membranes, primarily into skeletal muscle cells. Fatty acids, remaining bound to glycerol by the restoration of insulin inhibition of lipoprotein lipase, were now prevented from leaving fat cells. Glucose would again be expected to become the primary fuel of cellular metabolism.[25, 48]

The improvement in insulin sensitivity is reflected in the lower fasting insulins in the 5 patients with pre-treatment elevations of this measure (Figure 4A).

One point worth noting is the 120-minute blood insulin. Even when the GTT had become normal, with peak and AUC blood insulin in the same range as controls, the 120-minute blood insulin remained slightly elevated. In all controls the insulin level at 120 minutes was less than or equal to 19μIU/ml, whereas patients exhibited 120-minute insulin levels of at least 31μIU/ml, and 5 out of 9 patients showed levels greater than 80μIU/ml (Figure 4C).

Electrolytes — Changes Pre- to Post-Treatment: The pre-treatment 24-hour urine specimens showed a striking decrease from normal in the excretion of calcium, magnesium, and phosphorus.

In each instance a strong move to or toward normal was seen in the post-treatment 24-hour excretion. The same was found in "Case One," the patient who proved to have NIDDM and whose laboratory data are presented in detail elsewhere.

Glucose-Fatty Acid Cycle: Randle in 1963 proposed a competitive metabolism between glucose and FFA.[25] When available in adequate quantity, FFA are utilized by cells as their primary fuel; otherwise glucose is metabolized. As discussed above, the blood level of each is strongly influenced by insulin, although by different mechanisms. Prior to treatment the elevated level of FFA suggests these as the primary fuel of cellular metabolism, whereas after treatment, with the decreased availability of FFA, glucose assumes that role. Randle termed this the "glucose-fatty acid cycle."

Recent studies have sought to clarify the means by which FFA induce insulin resistance. Randle's original hypothesis was that increased cellular metabolism of FFA leads to accumulations of acetyl-CoA and of citrate, which, in turn, inhibit phosphofructokinase to cause increased intracellular glucose-6-PO_4.

More recently, based on lipid infusions together with a glucose-insulin clamp, evidence was found that FFA lead to insulin resistance by impairing the *membrane transport of glucose* rather than by interfering with its phosphorylation.[49] This conclusion was based on the finding in skeletal muscle cells of *decreased* intracellular glucose and *decreased* glucose-6-PO_4, whereas the mechanism originally proposed by Randle should have resulted in *elevated* cellular glucose and *elevated* glucose-6-PO_4. These same recent studies also demonstrated an approximately 50% reduction in muscle glycogen synthesis, in addition to a similar reduction in glucose oxidation.

Also found to correlate with insulin resistance was an increase in the saturated/unsaturated fatty acid ratio in muscle triglycerides, as well as the total level of muscle triglyceride.[50] Such an increase in saturated fatty acids at the expense of unsaturated fatty acids was previously reported in SCS patients, both in erythrocyte membranes and in plasma.[19]

Lipid Profile: In the early months of treatment, diet is of great help in suppressing Candida albicans. As many yeast cells as possible are killed with the safe drug, nystatin. Yeast cells that are beyond the reach of nystatin (e.g., sinuses, intracellular sites within cells of the deeper layers of the mucosae of the GI tract and vagina) are inhibited in their growth and toxin production by limiting their access to glucose molecules (sugars and starches). The beginning diet usually allows approximately 80 grams of carbohydrates per day. Once symptoms are controlled, the carbohydrate allowance is increased to 120-150 grams per day.

Patients who are overweight will utilize body fat to replace the carbohydrate calories removed from the diet. Patients who are at normal or subnormal weight will need to offset the calorie deficit (imposed by the temporary limitation of carbohydrate intake), with an increase in their intake of protein and fat calories; otherwise, they will become even thinner, or else the carbohydrate intake will have to be increased prematurely, before symptoms have been fully controlled.

To evaluate the effect of the increased fat intake, the lipid profile was followed in a large number of SCS patients. The changes in the various components of the lipid profile were analyzed at the end of the first year (Figure 11). This was chosen because thereafter carbohydrates would have been increased with a corresponding decrease in fat. The first year should give the best indication of any significant effect of the increased fat intake, particularly since this is the time when patients are the most conscientious about their diet.

Having followed many patients this way for 14 years, it has been noted that in many instances *improvement* has occurred in the lipid profile; it has never been necessary to discontinue the diet because of deterioration of the lipid profile. Thus we were not surprised by the improvement in the various components of the lipid profile, shown in Figure 11 (results of an analysis of 405 consecutive patients treated for SCS).

These findings suggest that interference with lipid chemistry may be one more effect (correctable) of the chronic release into the bloodstream of the many foreign substances produced by this fungus.

Insulin Resistance—Natural History: As noted earlier, in siblings of diabetic patients progression in the severity of insulin resistance may span decades, until often they too "become diabetic" as insulin resistance reaches that level of severity required for this diagnosis.

At the advanced stage of insulin resistance considered type II diabetes mellitus (i.e., either a fasting blood glucose >126 mg% or a 120-minute blood glucose >200 mg%), the blood insulin level often is higher than normal. It also may be low, even to the point that eventually insulin therapy is necessary, when the pancreatic islets can no longer supply the large amount of insulin necessary to compensate for the decreased sensitivity of tissues to the influence of this hormone. As also noted earlier, this same progression from mild to severe insulin resistance was seen when diabetes-prone obese monkeys were followed from birth to age 17 years.[23-24]

Patients in this study demonstrated the same spectrum of insulin resistance (Figure 2) from mild to severe seen over time in the siblings of diabetic patients and in obese diabetic monkeys. In fact, looking at this group of patients as a whole is almost like looking at the progression over many years of insulin resistance in the sibling of a diabetic patient, with the insulin resistance ranging from mild ("hyperinsulinism") to severe ("type II diabetes mellitus," "NIDDM").

In addition to the patient who proved to be diabetic ("Case One"), another patient had a pre-treatment 120-minute glucose of 194 mg% on the GTT, this just 6 mg% below the 120-minute 200 mg% level, agreed upon by convention, for the diagnosis of NIDDM. Striking improvement had occurred after 12 months treatment (Figure 8), both in her symptoms and in the insulin resistance.

Insulin is instrumental in regulating the blood level of both glucose and FFA. However, in contrast to the movement of FFA into the bloodstream from fat cells, the *entrance* of glucose into the bloodstream from the intestine is *independent* of regulation by insulin. Thus, insulin prevents dangerously high blood levels of each, although by different mechanisms—of FFA by inhibiting their entrance *into* the bloodstream, of glucose by promoting its exit *from* the bloodstream. The pancreas adjusts the amount of insulin released according to the amount of glucose being metabolized within the beta cells of the islets. As long as insulin sensitivity remains normal, glucose transport remains normally sensitive to insulin, plasma FFA are not elevated, and the GTT remains normal without the necessity for excessive insulin release.

Transport in the Nephron: Active glucose transport in the nephron is charged with conserving an extremely large amount of glucose, even when the blood sugar is normal. After transport across its luminal membrane into the nephron cell, and to prevent intracellular accumulation that would inhibit continuation of this initial step, glucose is transported by the Na^+-K^+ ATPase pump across the basolateral membrane of the cell, into the extracellular fluid, and ultimately into the renal vein. As noted elsewhere, the function of the Na^+-K^+ ATPase pump has been shown to be inhibited in states of increased membrane rigidity. This has been attributed to interference with the conformational change inherent in the function of this enzyme—an enzyme that is vital to every organ and for electrical conduction.

Insulin facilitates glucose conservation by stimulating its transport in the proximal tubule. Glycosuria occurring in these patients, even when the blood sugar is low and hence the glucose load light, is consistent with the concept of insulin resistance in the proximal tubule of the nephron. Treatment that corrected insulin resistance elsewhere, manifested as abnormal glucose tolerance and elevated plasma FFA, likewise was associated with a striking decrease or disappearance of glycosuria at these low blood glucose levels.

Thus, following relief of both local and generalized symptoms of SCS, insulin resistance was found to be relieved 1) in adipose cells, 2) in nephron cells, and 3) in skeletal muscle cells, the primary destination of glucose leaving the bloodstream.

CASE ONE

A woman 36 years of age presented with intractable yeast vaginitis, itching and discharge, dating from her first pregnancy, both recurring early in her second pregnancy. Eventually it became intractable. Contraceptive hormones (BCP) at age 36 led to hypertension and severe depression, both of which improved on discontinuing BCP. Associated symptoms included fatigue, alopecia, abdominal bloating, and alternating constipation and diarrhea. Highly significant diagnostically is the fact that the diarrhea had been aggravated repeatedly by antibiotics that at the same time had led to yeast vaginitis. Loss of memory and concentrating ability occurred intermittently, but depression was constant. Regular menstrual periods were heavy and associated with ten days of "severe" PMS; loss of libido had begun ten years earlier. Intolerance to inhaled chemicals was limited to tobacco smoke, but this was severe.

Relevant to these symptoms of chronic yeast infections were two episodes of rheumatic fever for which she received "many months" of antibiotic preventive therapy; no permanent valvular damage had been diagnosed. Also relevant is the family history strongly positive for diabetes.

Her pre-treatment GTT (Figure 3A) was diagnostic of NIDDM, with the 120-minute glucose at 201 mg% despite a 120-minute blood insulin of 610mIU/mL (approximately 10 times the level in control patients). She had become almost asymptomatic after 6 weeks treatment, including resumption of normal bowel function, PMS relief, and return to normal energy. A temporary relapse (vaginitis and diarrhea) occurred with antibiotic therapy for a dental problem.

At 6-months of treatment, bowel function was normal, energy was "fine," depression and PMS were absent, and she began noticing improvement in libido. Considerable improvement was seen at the time of the first repeat GTT (Figure 3B).

At 21 months she remained asymptomatic and the GTT was entirely normal with a maximum insulin in the same range as controls (Figure 3C.) In other words, there was no remaining indication whatsoever of the severe insulin resistance that had been present prior to treatment. The improvement could not be attributed to improvement in her obesity since the pre-treatment weight was 162 pounds. and at 21 months remained at 160 pounds.

When she discontinued treatment at 24 months, symptoms returned together with weight gain of 22 pounds. Diarrhea, vaginitis, and fatigue again cleared quickly with resumption of the anti-yeast program. Repeat GTT prior to resuming treatment is shown (Figure 3D). The insulin resistance had returned and was at approximately the level of severity seen after the first 6 months of treatment. She remained asymptomatic 4 months after resumption of treatment at 30 months (following 6 months off of treatment).

This case illustrates the fact that symptoms cannot be attributed to insulin resistance per se, defined in terms of glucose transport from the bloodstream. These patients become asymptomatic long before insulin sensitivity has returned to normal. This is consistent with the absence of symptoms in diabetic siblings despite insulin resistance that becomes progressively more severe over a span of many years.

INSULIN RESISTANCE

"Insulin resistance" may be defined as decreased sensitivity to insulin. More insulin than usual is required to elicit the same degree of response in one or more of the physiologic processes influenced by this hormone. Of these, the insulin-driven transport of glucose from plasma into cells has been the most intensively studied, normals having been established for the standard "glucose tolerance test" (GTT).

In its incipient stage, when defined in terms of glucose transport from blood, insulin resistance is seen simply as an increased amount of insulin required to maintain the glucose tolerance curve in the accepted normal range; this has been termed "hyperinsulinism." As insulin resistance progresses in severity, glucose tolerance becomes "impaired," meaning that at 120 minutes of a standard GTT the blood sugar level has failed to return approximately to the fasting level, often despite greatly increased amounts of insulin released into the bloodstream by the pancreas.

Though mild initially, impairment of the GTT may progress in severity so that, despite the release of ever higher amounts of insulin by the pancreas, the 120-minute glucose level continues to rise. By convention, agreed upon at the 1981 World Conference on Diabetes, when the 120-minute glucose is 200 mg% or higher, insulin resistance has reached the degree of severity that justifies the diagnosis of type II diabetes mellitus.

A highly important characteristic of insulin resistance is that it may vary from organ to organ. In fact, it has been stated that insulin resistance may be limited to a single organ, tissue, or even a single cell. If, over time, insulin resistance changes in severity in the different organs or even in the same organ, it might be anticipated that, in a given patient, the balance among the various symptoms would fluctuate accordingly.

Adding further to the complexity of understanding the long-term effects of insulin resistance is the relatively recent knowledge of the many additional pathways influenced by insulin. Chronically elevated blood levels of insulin, resulting from pancreatic compensation for the decreased response of glucose transport, should affect these other insulin-regulated processes. Various clinical patterns might be anticipated from 1) the degree to which resistance to insulin is shared by these other processes, 2) increased insulin stimulation of any process not sharing in the resistance to insulin, and 3) the extent to which the increased amount of insulin is able to compensate for such resistance in particular pathways, as when increased insulin is able to maintain normal glucose tolerance. Two examples illustrate the diverse clinical results that might ensue:

1) When insulin levels rise because of impaired sensitivity of the glucose response, stimulation of sodium reabsorption in the nephron is retained, that is, the stimulation by insulin of sodium reabsorption does not participate in insulin resistance. The resulting over-stimulation as a result of the elevated insulin levels may play a role in the etiology of hypertension, a condition characterized by insulin resistance.

2) As demonstrated in these patients, resistance to insulin inhibition of fatty acid release from triacylglyceride stores may or may not occur. Thus, many patients had elevated blood FFA levels, indicating resistance to insulin action in adipose cells; others had very low FFA levels, suggesting that in these patients the insulin resistance did not carry over to adipose cells so that lipolysis remained strongly inhibited by the high insulin levels.

Among the many actions of insulin, apart from regulation of glucose disposal, are the following: inhibition of excretion of sodium and uric acid, inhibition of platelet aggregation and lipolysis, vasodilation, hyperpolarization of membranes, sympathetic excitation, stimulation of corticotropin releasing factor, and stimulation of DNA and growth. A recent excellent review of this subject is available.[51] Varying degrees of resistance among these many processes influenced by insulin should result in varying combinations of pathophysiology, with corresponding variation in the patterns of resulting symptoms. Counter-regulatory responses would only add to the complexity of the situation.

Insulin and Memory: Of particular interest is the accumulating evidence that insulin may be involved in memory processes. Decreased short-term memory and concentrating ability is perhaps the most consistent generalized symptom in patients with

SCS; even young patients complain bitterly of this problem. Memory and concentrating ability return to normal with successful treatment of mucosal yeast infections. Further, evidence is mounting that insulin improves memory, even in patients with Alzheimer's disease.[52]

Insulin-Stimulated Membrane Transport: Relevant to the findings in the current study is the effect that increased membrane rigidity may have on functional responses of cells to insulin. This has been studied experimentally.

Insulin action includes mobilization to the cell membrane of insulin receptors stored inside the cell; functional responses thereafter are initiated by the binding of insulin to these receptors. When membranes were experimentally made more rigid by increases in the degree of saturation of their membrane-phospholipid fatty-acyl chains, insulin binding decreased significantly; insulin receptors in these cell membranes were reduced both in number and in their affinity for insulin.[53] Such inability of insulin to bind normally results in less than the expected functional responses of cells to a given amount of insulin, i.e., "insulin resistance." Shown to be less sensitive to the normal effect of insulin in such cells are membrane transport of glucose and amino acids, glycogen synthesis, and insulin-stimulated synthesis of RNA.

Type II Diabetes Mellitus and Candida Albicans: In the last 30 years there has been a striking increase (700%) in the incidence of this type of diabetes, also known as adult or non-insulin dependent diabetes mellitus (NIDDM). There has been no clue as to the cause other than possibly the increase in obesity in the general population.

About 1940 there began a steady increase in the prevalence of superficial candidiasis as represented by the reported increase in yeast vaginitis. Reports indicated as much as a 1500% increase in the incidence of vaginal yeast infections over the span of years that encompassed the introduction of the three principal modalities of treatment that are associated with increases in the incidence of yeast infections—antibiotics, contraceptive hormones, and steroids and other forms of immunosuppressant therapy.

In these patients with SCS, insulin resistance ranged from mild to severe and was corrected by treatment that cleared the superficial yeast infections. This suggests that this fungus may be an additional risk factor for NIDDM in genetically predisposed individuals and that the great increase in the incidence of chronic yeast infections may be a factor in the simultaneous increase in the incidence of NIDDM. It also suggests that better control of Candida albicans could prove useful in reducing the severe insulin resistance of type II diabetes mellitus (as in "Case One"). Finally, if these relationships hold, it means that these three great advances in medicine (antibiotics, steroids, and hormones) underlie the increase in NIDDM with the yeast Candida albicans serving as the intermediary.

It further suggests the possible incorrectness of the long-held view that chronic glycosuria is responsible for the frequent yeast vaginitis known to occur in diabetic women. It suggests instead that the reverse may be the case—that glycosuria is secondary to yeast-related insulin resistance in the nephron, as in the women reported in this study. Thus the yeast vaginitis would indicate that yeast is contributing to the insulin resistance of NIDDM.

Representative of the overall findings in these 53 women are the results in the patient with the most advanced degree of insulin resistance ("Case One"). She exhibited the same abnormalities found in the group as a whole, as well as the same decrease in insulin resistance following treatment.

An extremely important aspect of the impact of a chronic yeast infection is its effect on the immune system. Evidence of defective immune responses has been presented and confirmed in patients with chronic yeast infections.

One of the most interesting aspects of this subject concerns autoimmune disease.[19] Striking benefit clinically has accompanied the clearing of chronic yeast infections in a significant number of patients with certain of these conditions.[16] Among the patients in this study were 2 women who, in addition to chronic yeast infections, also had multiple sclerosis; they exhibited the same abnormalities found in the group as a whole, as well as the same decrease in insulin resistance following treatment.

Syndrome X (The Metabolic Syndrome): As the number of recognized risk factors for cardiovascular disease steadily increased, collectively they came to be known as "Syndrome X"; insulin resistance was an original component of this syndrome. Now included are elevated triglycerides, abdominal obesity, increased plasminogen activator inhibitor-1, elevated FFA, low HDL, high LDL, high VLDL, increased BMI (body mass index), low-normal serum creatinine, and insulin resistance. These various risk factors have been added to "Syndrome X" as, one by one, they have been shown to correlate with each other and with the cholesterol/HDL ratio. More recently "Syndrome X" has been referred to as "The Metabolic Syndrome."

Analysis of additional risk factors is underway in a much larger group of patients with chronic yeast infections. Based on changes pre-to-post in treated patients, there is suggestive evidence of the presence in these patients of additional components of Syndrome X. These include serum levels of creatinine, HDL, LDL, chol/HDL, and uric acid. (These studies will be presented at a later time.)

Summary

In the present study of 53 women with the superficial candidiasis syndrome, a number of abnormalities were found that offer a plausible explanation for symptoms of such general nature as seen in these patients. Resistance to the action of insulin was evidenced with respect to: 1) impaired glucose transport from blood into cells, 2) reduced insulin suppression of FFA release from adipose cells, and 3) impaired insulin-stimulated glucose transport in the proximal tubule of the nephron.

Potentially of great significance is the strong evidence of defective function in the nephron, particularly in its proximal tubule segment. Glucose was present in urine specimens at blood glucose levels far below that at which this should occur. Other than the syndrome of "congenital low renal threshold," urine should be virtually free of glucose at blood glucose levels below 180 mg%. In many of these patients glycosuria occurred at blood glucose levels well below 100 mg%, even at levels as low as 60-80 mg% (Figure 6A)!

Further evidence of impaired conservation in the nephron was provided by abnormalities in electrolyte excretion when measured in 24-hour urine specimens. In a condition that progresses in severity, often over many years, one might anticipate depletion of total body stores of electrolytes that move with glucose, if glucose reabsorption is impaired as in these patients. To evaluate this possibility, 24-hour urine specimens were obtained. The very low phosphorous excretion and diminished magnesium excretion suggest maximum conservation efforts by the body, in turn suggesting diminished total body stores of these minerals. As symptoms disappeared with treatment of the chronic yeast infections, the strong move to or toward normal in the excretion of these electrolytes suggests repletion of body stores.

Lipid Profile: To determine whether the elements of the lipid profile were being altered in patients with chronic candidiasis, as well as to monitor the changes with treatment, the lipid profile has been followed in a large series of patients on long-term treatment.

The results are shown in Figure 11. There occurred statistically significant improvement in each component of the lipid profile. Thus it seems that the high carbohydrate diet, eaten by these patients prior to treatment, is more detrimental than the somewhat higher fat diet necessitated by the need to reduce carbohydrates in bringing this yeast under control.

Further, it allays concern that the increase in fat in proportion to carbohydrate would lead to changes in the lipid profile that might be harmful to the arteries.

SUMMARY AND CONCEPTS

Candida albicans is a fungus that is considered part of the "normal flora" that live on skin and on the mucous membranes of the vagina and gastrointestinal tract. Its growth is strongly stimulated by three of the greatest advancements in treatment in modern medicine—antibiotics, "birth control pills," and cortisone.

Candida albicans has been found to release into the human bloodstream a large number of substances that include toxins, enzymes, and other foreign proteins, sufficient in number to cause production by the immune system of 79 antibodies that react with this yeast. Very little is known about the long-term effects of these substances, but one effect that has been demonstrated is suppression of the immune system, i.e., immunologic tolerance (immunologic paralysis)—a weakening of the immune system.

The studies reported herein found a number of abnormalities in blood and urine, all of which were corrected by treatment that, based on disappearance of the local symptoms, eliminates the fungal invasion that had occurred in one or more of the superficial surfaces of the body. It is reasonable to assume that, once deprived of access to the bloodstream, Candida albicans is unable to continue releasing into the human bloodstream the large quantities of substances that had led to these biochemical abnormalities and their resultant symptoms.

This too allows the immune system to recover from the immunosuppression that had been caused by these yeast products. There is relief of local symptoms at the sites of mucosal colonization in the vagina and gastrointestinal tract; but, most importantly, symptoms are also alleviated that had resulted from the abnormalities in biochemical and physiologic processes induced (presumably) by this large array of toxins and foreign proteins that had been fed into the bloodstream from the sites of mucosal invasion.

Local symptoms at the sites of mucosal invasion include vaginal itching and/or discharge; upper gastrointestinal tract "heartburn" and/or nausea; and colon symptoms of "irritable bowel syndrome" that include excess gas and bloating, and abnormal bowel function—either diarrhea or constipation, or alternating diarrhea and constipation—and at times rectal itching. Significant in the history is aggravation of diarrhea by antibiotics; in women this often coincides with induction of yeast vaginitis.

The "general symptoms" described by these patients point to interference with various functions—energy metabolism, the emotional as well as the intellectual functions of the brain, hormone function, and intolerance to environmental substances such as fragrances, pesticides, cleansers, and exhaust fumes. The symptoms that result include severe lethargy (energy metabolism); inappropriate anxiety and depression, insomnia, panic attacks, great difficulty with short-term memory and concentration (brain); impotence and acne in men (hormones); and in women severe hormone (menstrual) problems that may include acne, PMS, bleeding abnormalities, decreased libido, sterility or frequent miscarriages (hormones); and from environment chemicals, such symptoms as weakness, fainting, and paresthesias.

Further, muscle and joint pains are common, as are "conventional" allergies that include chronic urticaria, asthma, migraine headaches, and nasal and sinus symptoms.

There is almost always a pathological craving for glucose molecules, i.e., sugars and starches. This led to the choice of glucose tolerance studies to investigate this condition. Insulin resistance was found, blood glucose failing to enter cells normally in response to elevated blood insulin levels. Such resistance in the response to insulin varied from mild to severe, one patient's blood sugar elevation actually meeting the criteria for the diagnosis of NIDDM (non-insulin dependent diabetes mellitus) despite a blood insulin level 10 times that of controls ("Case One" presented in detail).

Elevated free fatty acids (FFA) indicated that fat cells too were resistant to the normal suppression by insulin of the release of FFA into the bloodstream. This also indicated the utilization of more FFA in place of glucose for cell metabolism.

Insulin resistance in the nephron may be the reason for the defective conservation of glucose (and probably electrolytes) by the kidney, much sugar being found in the urine of these patients, even at very low blood-sugar levels.

With treatment, additional observations included improvement in the various components of the lipid profile.

The patient who was diabetic ("Case One") was the only one found to have an elevated blood level of DHEA-S, hers being 701 against a normal of 35 to 430 (mcg/dL). This strongly suggests resistance in the adrenal glands to the normal suppressing effect of insulin on the release of DHEA-S, again despite the fact that in this patient the blood level of insulin reached 10 times that of controls during the GTT.

Worthy of special emphasis is a condition experienced by many women, one that is alleviated by treatment of SCS. This problem is that of urinary burning, frequency, and urgency that may last for years. Unfortunately antibiotics, almost always used repeatedly in an effort to correct these symptoms, only aggravate and prolong the problem. These symptoms disappear coincident with those in the vagina.

As the yeast is brought under control with appropriate treatment, improvement in insulin resistance and in all elements of the lipid profile (including triglycerides) relates Candida albicans to the "Metabolic Syndrome" (Syndrome X), and thus to the risk of cardiovascular disease. To repeat, these changes occurred despite the fact that the low carbohydrate diet necessitated an increase in fat consumption. Long-term follow-up of a large number of subjects will be necessary to evaluate this possibility.

Insulin resistance is the hallmark of type II diabetes. Since this was present in all degrees of severity in these patients, it strongly suggests that Candida albicans may at least be an aggravating factor in this condition. There was striking disappearance of all evidence of NIDDM in the patient reported as "Case One," in whom there was a strong family history of diabetes. After 21 months of treatment her 120-minute GTT was entirely normal, whereas prior to treatment her 120-minute blood glucose was 201 mg%, despite a simultaneous blood insulin of 610mIU—10 times the amount of insulin released in controls.

Did Candida albicans cause the severe insulin resistance of NIDDM in this genetically susceptible individual? The normal glucose tolerance test after 21 months of treatment of this yeast suggests this possibility. When she discontinued treatment after 25 months, return of the pre-treatment symptoms was accompanied by return of the insulin resistance; after 6 months off treatment, this was then at approximately the same degree of severity as had been found after 6 months of treatment.

The striking increase in the incidence of type II diabetes in the last 30-40 years has coincided with the great increase in the frequency of superficial yeast infections. While it is well known that correlation does not prove cause and effect, the insulin resistance found in patients with intractable yeast infections may at least be an aggravating factor in NIDDM.

BIBLIOGRAPHY

1. Kirkpatrick CH. Mitogen and antigen-induced lymphocyte responses in patients with infectious diseases. In: Oppenheim JJ, Rosinstreich, eds. Mitogens and Immunology. New York: Academic Press, 1976:239–665.

2. Kirkpatrick CH, Rich RR, Bennett JE. Chronic mucocutaneous candidiasis: model-building in cellular immunity, Ann Intern Med. 1971 Jun; 74(6): 955–78.

3. Fidel PL Jr, Lynch ME, et al. Systemic cell-mediated immune reactivity in women with recurrent vulvovaginal candidiasis. J Infect Dis. 1993, Dec; 168(6): 1458–65.

4. Witkin SS. Defective immune responses in patients with recurrent candidiasis. Infections in Medicine 1985.

5. Witkin SS, Yu IR, Ledger WJ. Inhibition of Candida albicans-induced lymphocyte proliferation by lymphocytes and sera from women with recurrent vaginitis. Am J Obstet Gynecol. 1983 Dec 1; 147(7): 809–11.

6. Vardinon N, Segal E. Suppressive action of Candida albicans on the immune response in mice. Exp Cell Biol. 1979; 47(4): 275–80.

7. Rogers TJ, Balish E. Suppression of lymphocyte blastogenesis by Candida albicans. Clin Immunol & Immunopathol. 1978 Jul; 10(3): 298–305.

8. Rogers TJ, Balish E. Immunity to Candida albicans. Microbiol Rev. 1980 Dec; 44(4): 660–82

9. Iwata K, Uchida K. Cell-Mediated immune responses of mice in experimental Candida infection: the influence of canditoxin on activity of lymphoid cells. Jpn J Med Sci Biol. 1978 Apr 31(2): 195–7.

10. Axelsen NH. Analysis of human Candida precipitins by quantitative immunoelectrophoresis: a model for analysis of complex microbial antigen-antibody systems. Scand J Immunol. 1976; 5(3): 177–90.

11. Iwata K. Toxins produced by Candida albicans. Contrib Microbiol Immunol. 1977, 4: 77–85.

12. Iwata K. Fungal toxins as a parasitic factor responsible for the establishment of fungal infections. Mycopathologia 1978 Dec 18 (1-3); 65:141–54.

13. Edwards JE Jr, Lehrer RI, et al. Severe candidal infections: Clinical perspective, immune defense mechanisms, and current concepts of therapy. Ann Int Med. 1978 July; 8(1): 91–106.

14. Truss CO, Truss CV, Cutler RB. Generalized symptoms in women with chronic yeast vaginitis: treatment with nystatin, diet and immunotherapy versus nystatin alone. J Advancement Med 1992; 5(3):139–75.

15. Dismukes WE, Wade JS, et al. A randomized double-blind trial of nystatin therapy for the candidiasis hypersensitivity syndrome. N. Engl J Med. 1990; 323(25): 1717–23.

16. Truss CO. The Missing Diagnosis, 2nd Ed. Birmingham, AL. The Missing Diagnosis, Inc. 1986.

17. Truss CO. Tissue injury induced by Candida albicans: mental and neurologic manifestations. J Orthomolecular Psychiatry 1978; 7: 17–37.

18. Wade JC, Schimpff SC, et al. A comparison of trimethoprimsulfamethoxazole plus nystatin with gentamicin plus nystatin in the prevention of infections in acute leukemia. N Engl J Med. 1981 Apr 30; 304(18): 1057–62.

19. Truss CO. Metabolic abnormalities in patients with chronic candidiasis: the acetaldehyde hypothesis. J Orthomolecular Psychiatry 1984; 13: 66–93.

20. Keston AS. Specific colorimetric enzymatic analytical reagents for glucose. Abstract of papers 129th Meeting ACS Dallas, Texas 1956.

21. Trendor P. Determination of glucose in blood using glucose oxidase with an alternative oxygen acceptor. Ann Clin Bio Chem 1969; 6–24.

22. Truss Co, Truss CV, Cutler RB, Llabre MM. Letter to editor. N Engl J Med 1991; 1592.

23. Hansen BC. Pathophysiology of obesity-associated type II diabetes (NIDDM): implications from longitudinal studies of non-human primates. Nutrition 1989 Jan-Feb; 5(1): 48–50.

24. Pender C, Ortmeyer HK, et al. Elevated plasma cell membrane glycoprotein levels and diminished insulin receptor auto-phosphorylation in obese, insulin-resistant rhesus monkeys. Metabolism 2002 Apr; 51(4): 465–70.

25. Randle PJ, Hales CN, Garland PB, Newsholme EA. The glucose-fatty acid cycle: its role in insulin sensitivity and the metabolic disturbances of diabetes mellitus. Lancet. 1963 Apr 13; 1: 785–89.

26. Farias RN, Bloj B, Morero RD, et al. Regulation of allosteric membrane-bound enzymes through changes in memrane lipid composition. Biochim Biophys Acta. 1975 Jun 30; 415(2): 231–51.

27. Muriel P, Mourelle M. Characterization of membrane fraction lipid composition and function of cirrhotic rat liver. J Hepatol. 1992 Jan;14(1):16–21.

28. Owen JS, McIntyre N, Gillett MPT. Lipoproteins, cell membranes and cellular functions. TIS 1984; 238–42.

29. Sandermann H Jr. Regulation of membrane enzymes by lipids. Biochim Biophys Acta. 1978 Sep 29; 515(3): 209–37.

30. Vickers JD, Rathbone MP. The effect of membrane cholesterol depletion upon erythrocyte membrane-bound enzymes. Can J Biochem. 1979 Sep; 57(9): 1144–52.

31. Kaduce TL, Awad AB, et al. Effect of fatty acid saturation on α-aminoisobutyric acid transport in Ehrlich ascites cells. J Biol Chem 1977 Oct 10; 252(19): 6624–30.

32. Im WB, Deutchler JT, Spector AA. Effects of membrane fatty acid composition on sodium-independent phenylalanine transport in Ehrlich cells. Lipids. 1979 Dec; 14(12): 1003–8.

33. Melchior DL, Czech MP. Sensitivity of the adipocyte D-glucose transport system to membrane fluidity in reconstituted vesicles. J Biol Chem. 1979 Sep 25; 254:8744–47.

34. Hirata F, Axelrod J. Enzymatic methylation of phosphatidyl ethanolamine increases erythrocyte membrane fluidity. Nature. 1978 Sep 21; 275(5677): 219–20.

35. Boelsteril UA, Rakhit G, Balaza T. Modulation by S-adenosyl-L-methionine of hepatic Na^+, K^+-ATPase, membrane fluidity, and bile flow in rats with ethinyl estradiol- induced cholestasis. Hepatology. 1983 Jan-Feb; 3(1): 12–17.

36. Kimelberg HK. Alterations in phospholipid-dependent (Na^+ + K^+)-ATPase activity due to lipid fluidity. Biochim Biophys Acta. 1975 Nov 17; 413(1): 143–56.

37. Leoni S, Luly P, Mangiantini MT, Spagnuolo S. Effect of free fatty acids and cholesterol in vitro on liver plasma membrane-bound enzymes. Experientia. 1982 Jan 15; 38(1): 102–4.

38. Kimelberg HK, Papahadjopoulos D. Effects of phospholipid acyl chain fluidity, phase transitions, and cholesterol on (Na^+ + K^+)-stimulated adenosine triphosphatase. J Biol Chem 1974 Feb 25; 249(4): 1071–80.

39. Raison JK, Lyons JM, Thomson WW. The influence of membranes on the temperature-induced changes in the kinetics of some respiratory enzymes of mitochondria. Arch Biochem Biophys. 1971 Jan; 142(1): 83–90.

40. Owen JS, Gillett MP. Plasma lipids, liproteins and cell membranes. Biochem Soc Trans. 1983 Aug; 11(4): 336–39.

41. Watala C, Winocour PD. The relationship of chemical modification of membrane proteins and plasma lipoproteins to reduced membrane fluidity of erythrocytes from diabetic subjects. Eur J Clin Chem Clin Biochem. 1992 Sep; 30(9): 513–19.

42. Watala C. Altered structural and dynamic properties of blood cell membranes in diabetes mellitus. Diabet Med. 1993 Jan-Feb; 10(1): 13–20.

43. Kamada T. Yamashita T, et al. Dietary sardine oil increases erythrocyte membrane fluidity in diabetic patients. Diabetes. 1986 May; 35(5): 604–11.

44. Coleman R. Membrane-bound enzymes and membrane ultrastructure. Biochim Biophys Acta. 1973 Apr 3; 300(1): 1–30.

45. Kinnunen PK. On the principles of functional ordering in biological membranes. Chem Phys Lipids. 1991 Mar; 57(2-3): 375–99.

46. Cooper RA. Abnormalities of cell-membrane fluidity in the pathogenesis of disease. Seminars in Medicine of the Beth Israel Hospital, Boston. N Engl J Med. 1977 Aug 18; 297(7): 371–7.

47. Schachter D. Fluidity and function of hepatocyte plasma membranes. Hepatology. 1984 Jan-Feb; 4(1): 140–51.

48. Randle PJ, Priestman DA, Mistry S, Halsall A. Mechanisms modifying glucose oxidation in diabetes mellitus. Diabetologia. 1994 Sep; 37 Suppl 2: S155–61.

49. Dresner A, Laurent D, et al. Effects of free fatty acids on glucose transport and IRS-1-associated phosphatidylinositol 3-kinase activity. J Clin Invest. 1999 Jan; 103(2): 253–259.

50. Manco M, Mingrone C, et al. Insulin resistance directly correlates with increased saturated fatty acids in skeletal muscle triglycerides. Metabolism. 2000 Feb; 49(2): 220–224.

51. Ferrannini E, Galvan AQ, et al. Insulin: new roles for an ancient hormone. Eur J Clin Invest. 1999 Oct; 29(10): 842–52.

52. Craft S, Aschana S, et al. Enhancement of memory in Alzheimer disease with insulin and somatostatin, but not glucose. Arch Gen Psychiatry. 1999 Dec; 56(12):1135–40.

53. Gould RJ, Ginsberg BH, Spector AA. Lipid effects on the binding properties of a reconstituted insulin receptor. J Biol Chem. 1982 Jan; 257(1): 477–84.

FIGURES AND TABLES

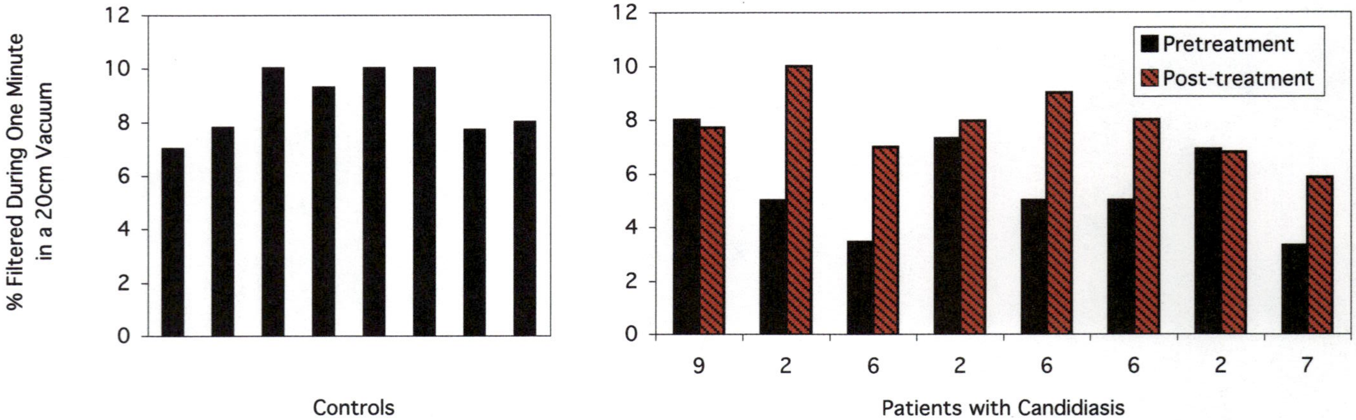

Figure 1. Red Blood Cell Filtration
RBC filtration rates of eight healthy adults as compared with the filtration rates of eight patients with candidiasis. Solid bars represent values of controls and of patients before treatment. Hatched bars represent values of patients after treatment. Duration of treatment in months is shown under each pre- and post-treatment pair.

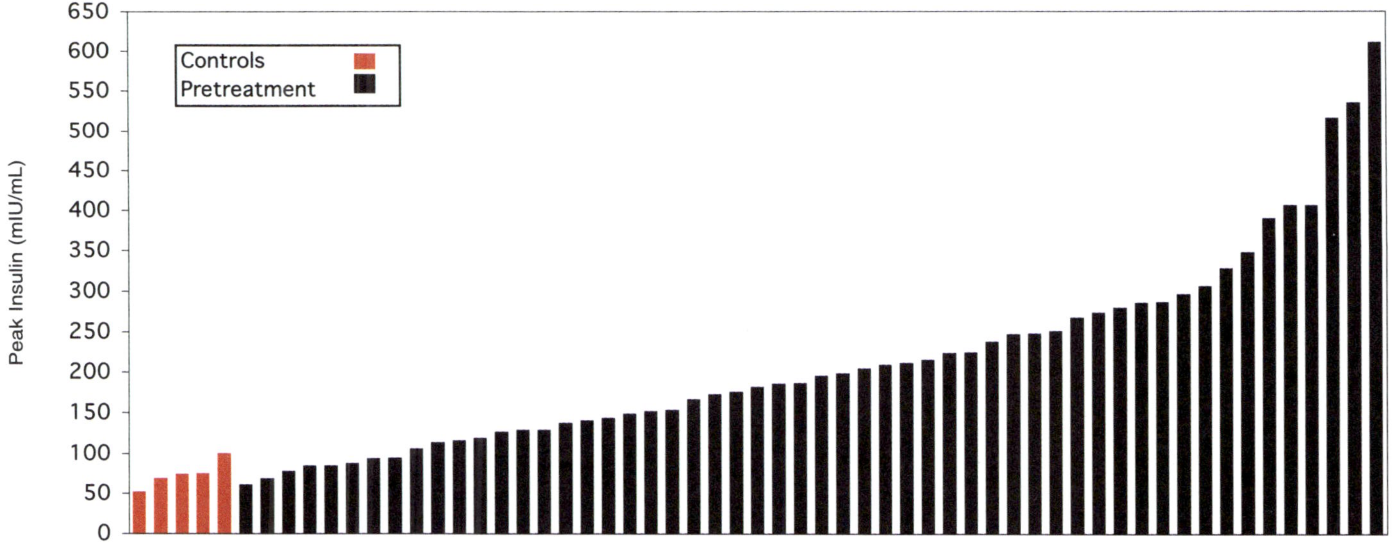

Figure 2. Pretreatment Peak Insulin Values
Peak blood insulin levels during glucose tolerence tests are shown for five controls and fifty-two patients with candidiasis (prior to treatment).

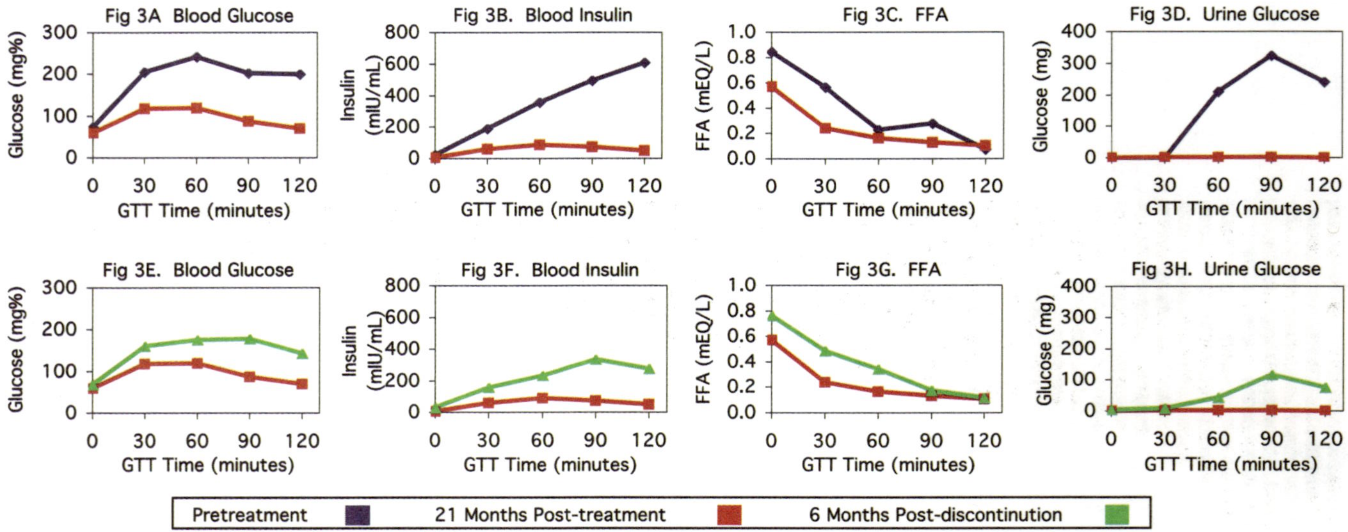

Figure 3. Case One, GTT Results Compared
Figures A through D show pretreatment and 21 month post-treatment results. Blood & urine glucose, insulin, and free fatty acids all showed marked improvement after treatment for candida albicans. Figures E through H show the 21 month post-treatment results compared to results at 30 months, 6 months after discontinuing treatment. Significant regression is seen in each component after only six months without treatment.

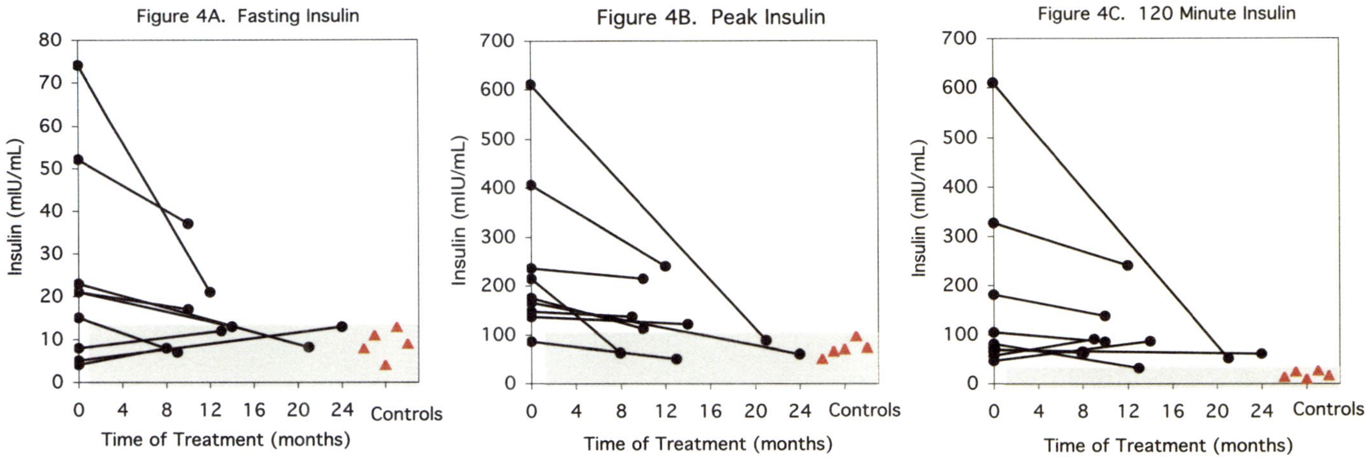

Figures 4A, 4B, and 4C. Insulin Levels During 2 Hour GTT
Fasting, peak, and 120 minute insulin levels are shown for 9 female candida patients and 5 controls. Black lines represent the change in insulin levels for the nine patients from pretreatment to post-treatment. Insulin levels for controls are shown in red. Each subject with elevated pretreatment fasting insulin showed improvement after treatment. Each patient also showed improvement (reduction) in peak insulin levels. Most patients showed improvement in 120 minute insulin levels as well; however all patients remained above the level of the controls.

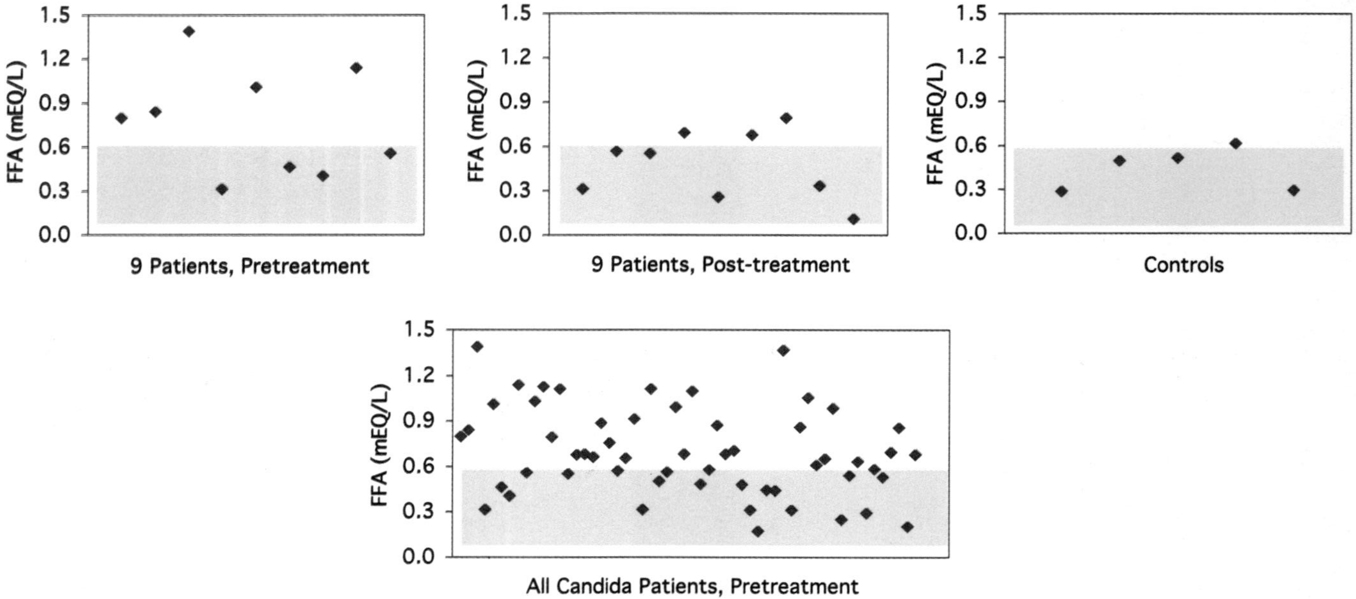

Figure 4D. Fasting Free Fatty Acids (FFA)
Free fatty acid levels shown for controls, all pretreatment candida patients, and the nine female candida patients for which pre- and post-treatment results were available. Shaded gray areas represent the normal range.

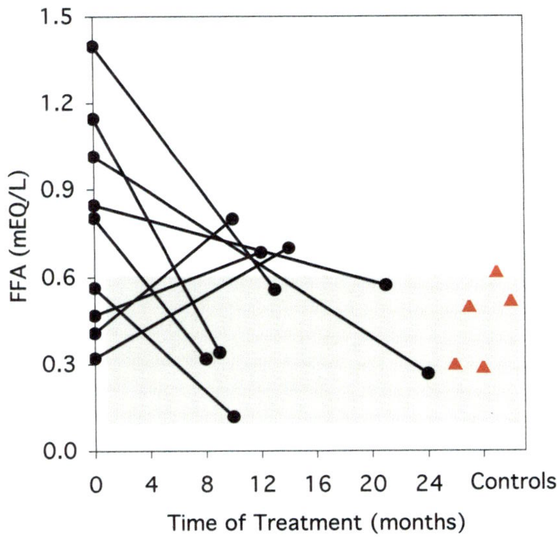

Figure 4E. Fasting Free Fatty Acids (FFA)
Fasting free fatty acid levels are shown for nine candida patients and five controls. Black lines represent the change in FFA levels for the nine patients subsequent to treatment for candida. Fasting FFA levels for the controls are shown in red. All patients with elevated pretreatment FFA fell into the normal range subsequent to treatment for candida.

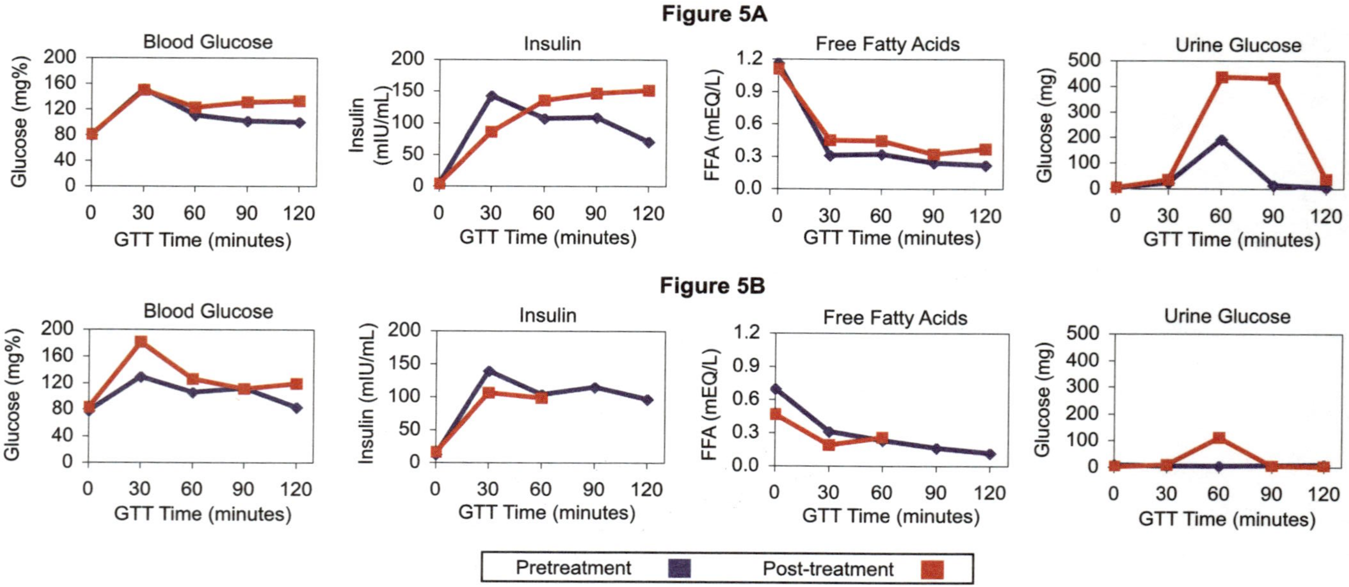

Figure 5A and 5B. Comparisons for Two Patients on Treatment Without Diet
Comparison of pre- and post-treatment GTT studies are shown for two patients who did not adhere to the low carbohydrate and low yeast diet, but were treated with nystatin and immunotherapy injections. Post-treatment results for the patients in Figures 5A and 5B were taken after 9 months and 8 months of treatment, respectively.

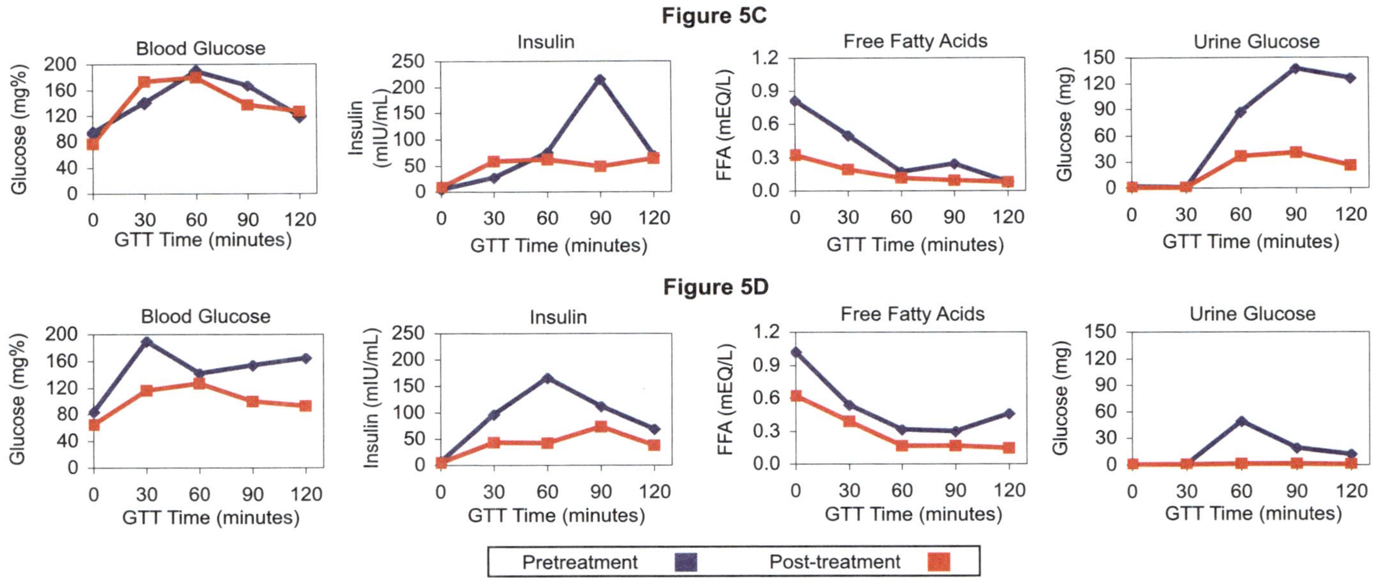

Figure 5C and 5D. Comparisons for Two Patients on Treatment Without Immunotherapy Injections
Comparison of pre- and post-treatment GTT studies are shown for two patients who were treated with nystatin and restricted diet, but who were not treated with immunotherapy injections. Post-treatment results shown for the patients in Figures 5C and 5D were taken after 8 months and 24 months of treatment, respectively.

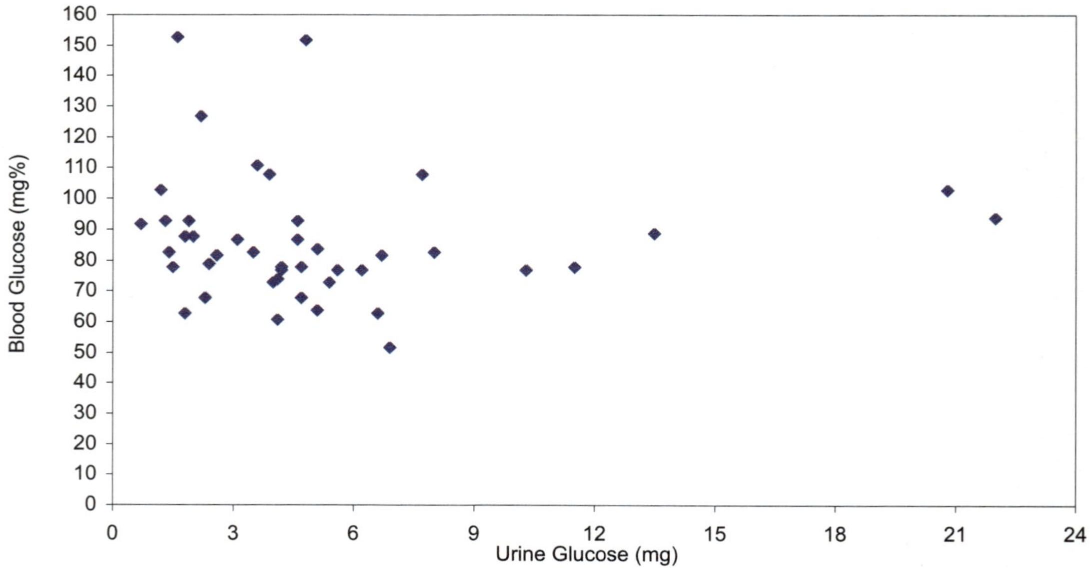

Figure 6A. Glycosuria in 43 Female Candida Patients
The lowest blood glucose level at which glucose was detected in the urine is shown for 43 patients prior to treatment for candida albicans. Note that 35 out of 43 patients showed glycosuria at blood glucose levels of 95mg% or lower, with five patients exhibiting glycosuria at blood glucose levels of 65mg% or lower.

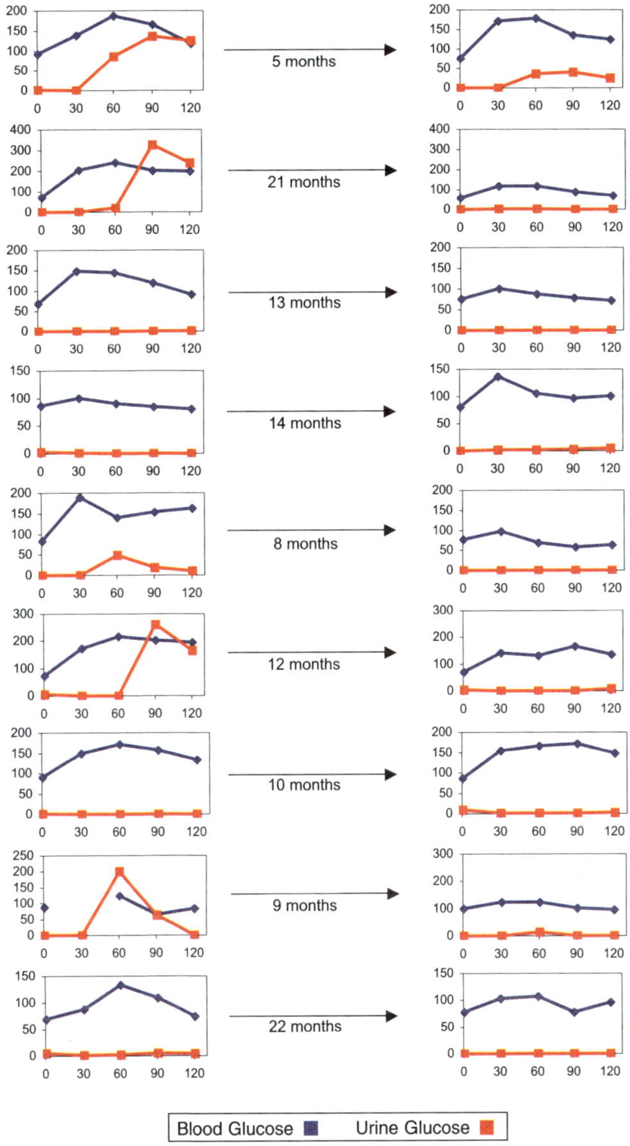

Figure 6B. Blood and Urine Glucose
Blood glucose (in mg%) and urine glucose (in total mg) are shown for nine patients who were treated for candidiasis. Values for each were recorded during pre- and post-treatment 120 minute GTT studies. The left column shows glucose values before treatment, and the right column shows post-treatment values. Duration of treatment is shown for each patient.

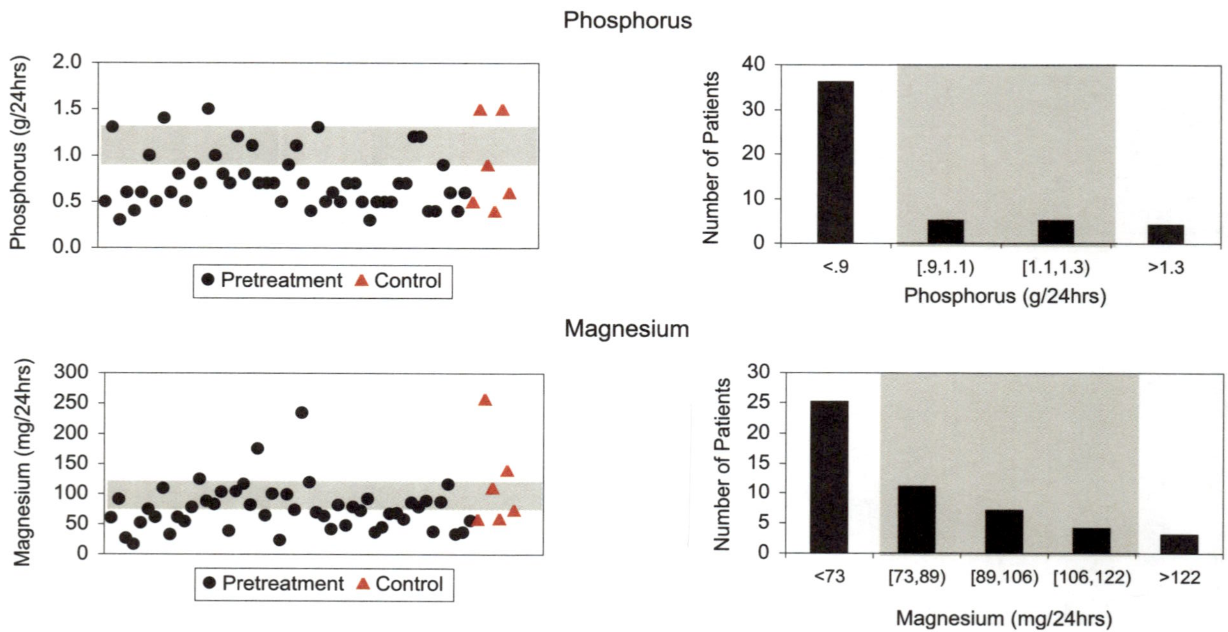

Figure 7A. Pre-treatment 24 Hour Urine Electrolytes
Phosphorus and magnesium levels recorded in 24 hour urine excretion are shown for 6 controls subjects and 50 female candida patients prior to treatment. The distributions of patient electrolyte levels are shown in histograms to the right. Gray shaded areas represent the normal range.

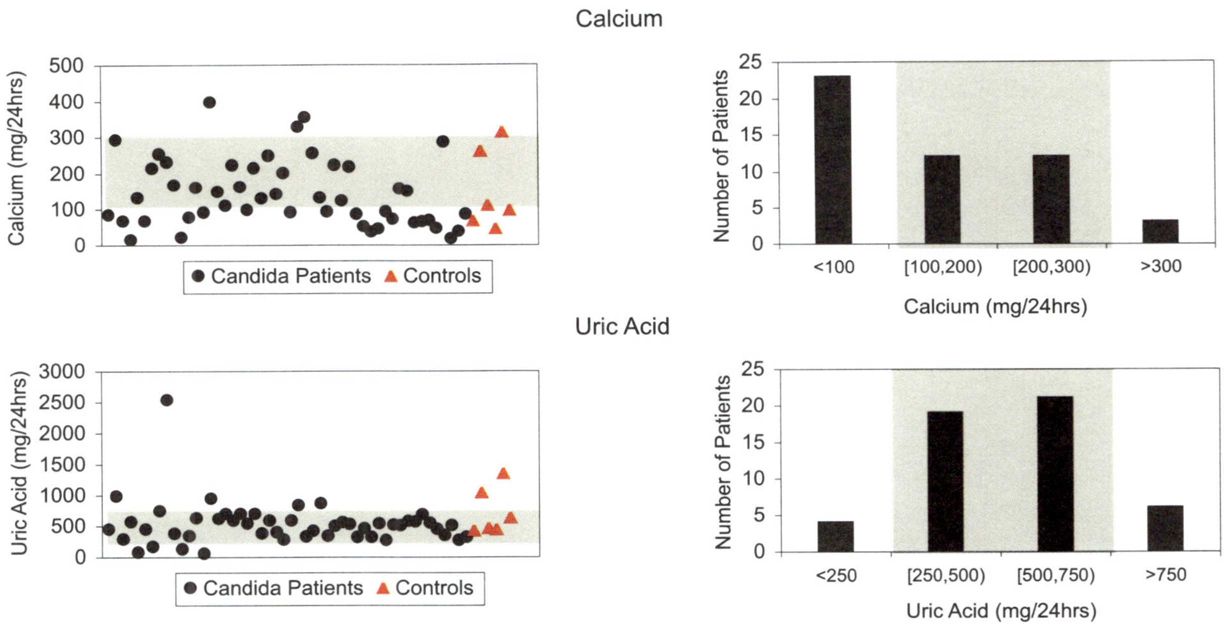

Figure 7B. Pre-treatment 24 Hour Urine Electrolytes
Calcium and uric acid levels recorded in 24 hour urine excretion are shown for 6 controls subjects and 50 female candida patients prior to treatment. The distributions of patient electrolyte levels are shown in histograms to the right. Gray shaded areas represent the normal range.

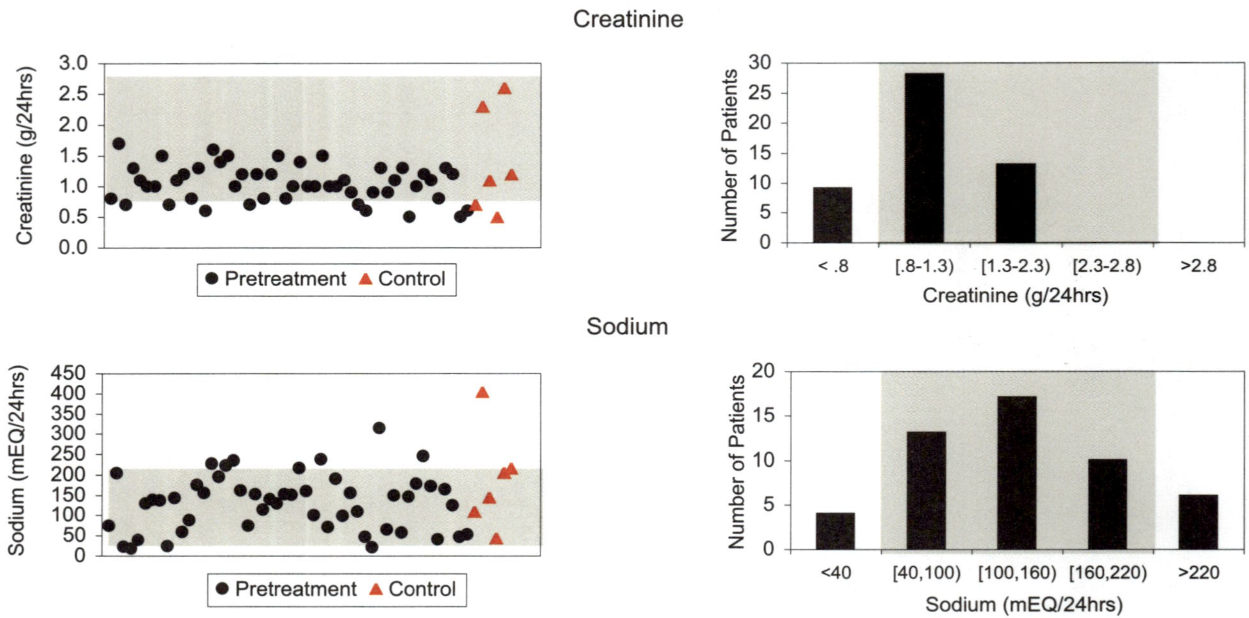

Figure 7C. Pre-treatment 24 Hour Urine Electrolytes
Creatinine and sodium levels recorded in 24 hour urine excretion are shown for 6 controls subjects and 50 female candida patients prior to treatment. The distributions of patient electrolyte levels are shown in histograms to the right. Gray shaded areas represent the normal range. Note that the insulin resistance with respect to glucose transport does not apply to the influence of insulin on the Na+-K+ ATPase pump and the transport of sodium in the renal proximal tubule.

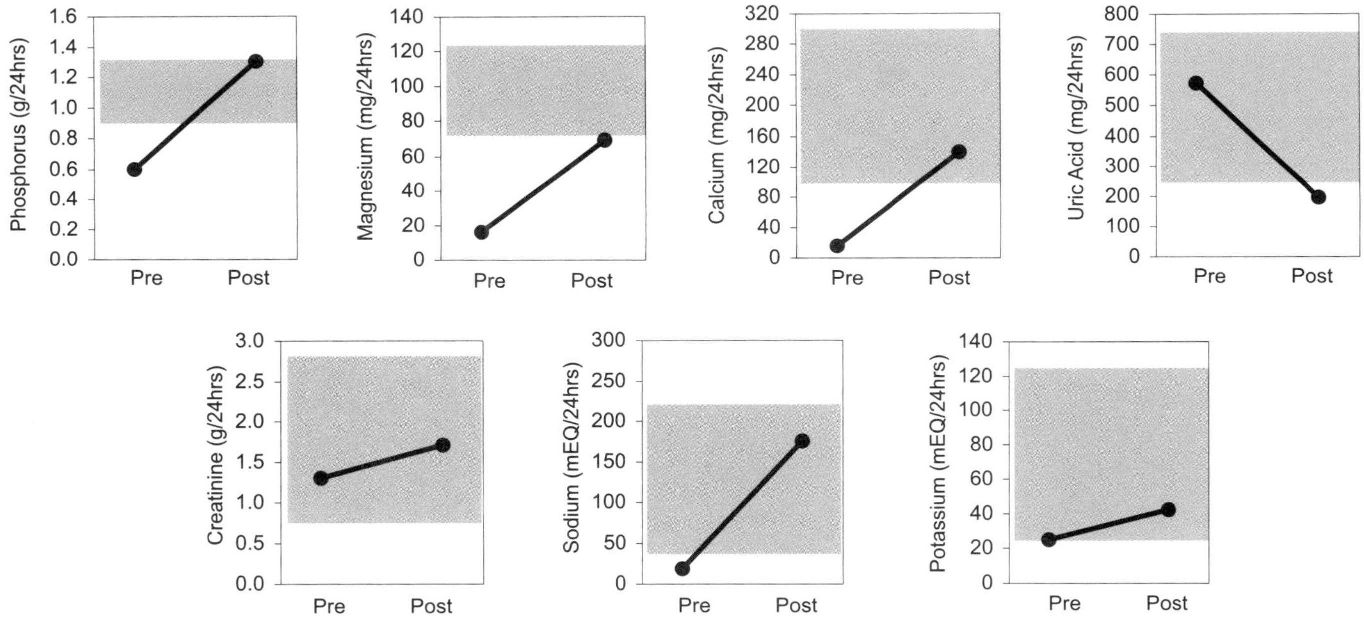

Figure 7D. Case One, 24 Hour Urine Electrolytes
Electrolyte levels recorded in pre- and post-treatment 24 hour urine excretion are shown for Case One. Post-treatment results were taken after six months of treatment. Gray shaded areas represent the normal range.

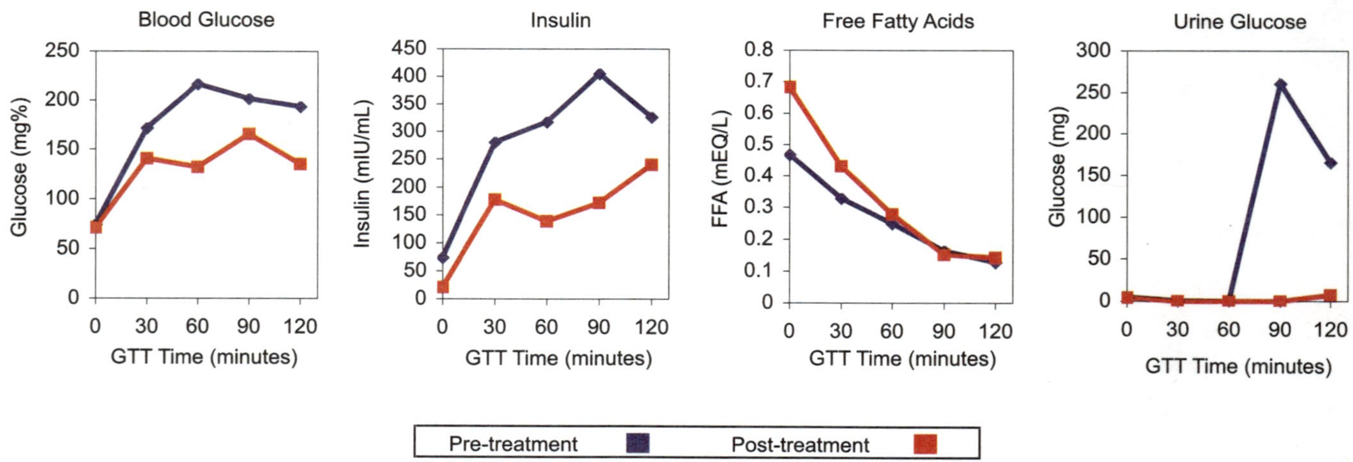

Figure 8. GTT Study Comparison
Pre-treatment and 12 month post-treatment GTT result comparisons are shown for a patient with a pre-treatment 120-minute blood glucose level of 194 mg%. Significant improvements were seen in the patient's glucose and insulin levels after one year of treatment for Candida albicans.

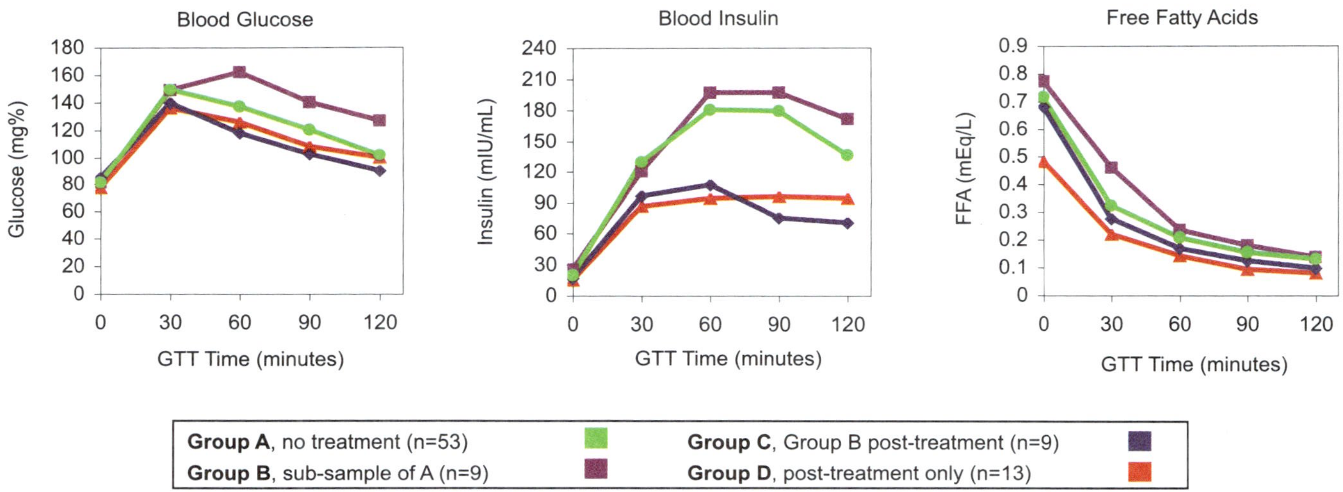

Figure 9. Pre- and Post- Treatment Female Candida Patient Groups Compared
Group A consists of pre-treatment GTT studies conducted on 53 patients. Group B is a subgroup of Group A, comprised of nine patients for whom post-treatment GTTs were available, and who followed the entire treatment protocol of diet, nystatin, and injections. Group C shows post-treatment studies on the nine full treatment patients of Group B. Group D consists of 13 patients with the same symptoms and treatment as the 9 patients of Group B, but who did not complete GTT studies prior to treatment. It was felt that these patients would reflect what might be expected of Group C patients after several years of treatment.

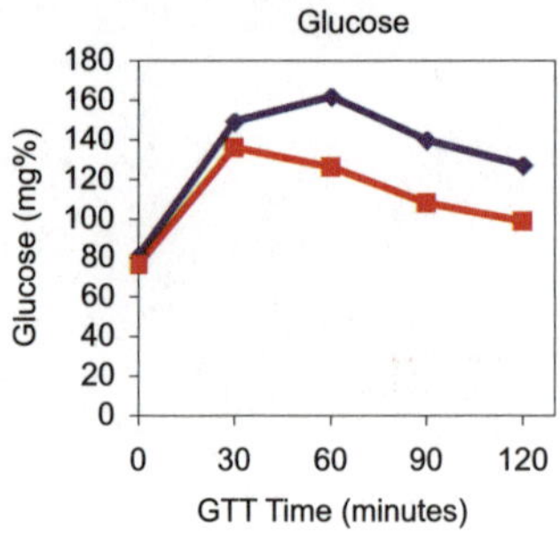

GTT time (min)	0	30	60	90	120
avg pretrt (mg%)	81	149	162	140	127
avg posttrt (mg%)	77	136	126	108	99
difference (mg%)	4	13	36	36	27

mean diff. 22
st.dev. 12
SEm 4
diff. is significant, p<.005, 1-tail

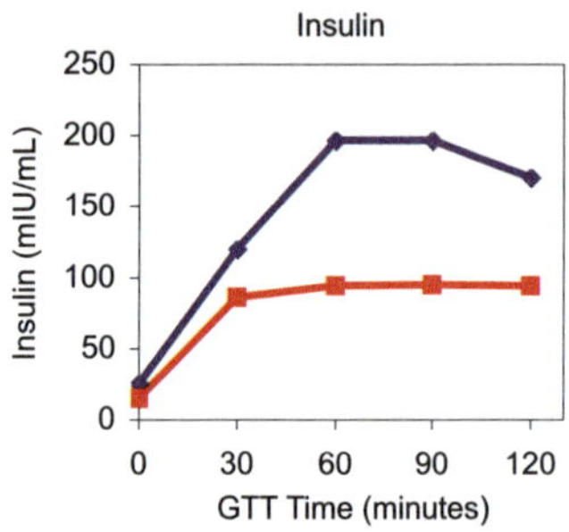

GTT time (min)	0	30	60	90	120
avg pretrt (mIU/mL)	25	120	197	197	171
avg posttrt (mIU/mL)	15	86	94	95	94
difference (mIU/mL)	10	34	103	101	78

mean diff. 65
st.dev. 37
SEm 17
diff. is significant, p<.01, 1-tail

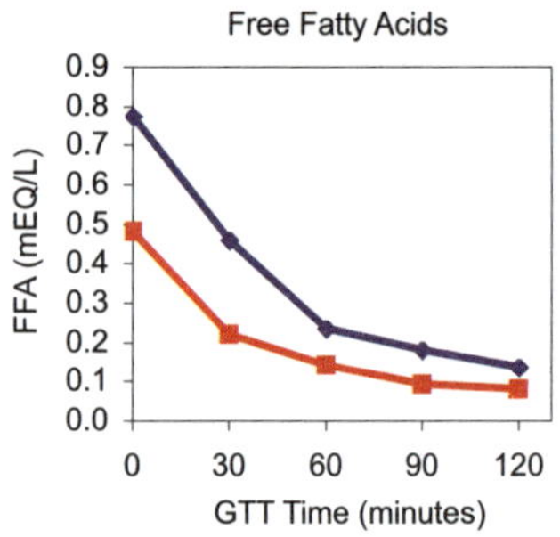

GTT time (min)	0	30	60	90	120
avg pretrt (mEQ/L)	0.774	0.459	0.235	0.181	0.137
avg posttrt (mEQ/L)	0.483	0.221	0.143	0.094	0.081
difference (mEQ/L)	0.29	0.238	0.092	0.086	0.056

mean diff. 0.153
st.dev. 0.093
SEm 0.047
diff. is significant, p<.015, 1-tail

Pretreatment ■ Post-treatment ■

Figure 10. Pre- and Post- Treatment GTT Results
Comparison of pre- and post-treatment average GTT results are shown for nine patients with full treatment for candidiasis. Note that glucose, insulin, and free fatty acid averages improved significantly at each sampling time subsequent to treatment.

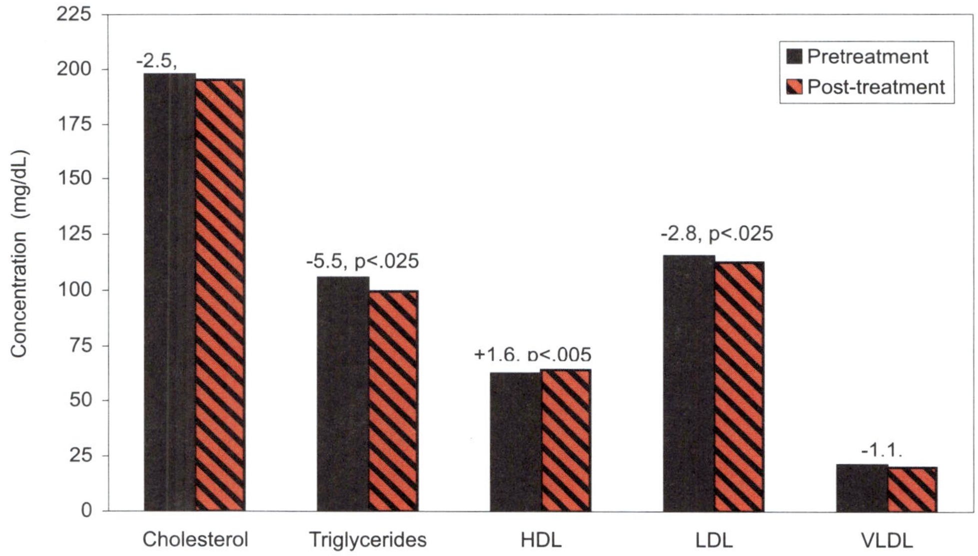

Figure 11. Lipid Profile Comparison
Average change in lipid profile components after 9-15 months of treatment are shown for 405 consecutive SCS patients. Numbers above each component reflect the absolute numerical change and the statistical significance calculated by correlated t-test of differences.

Table 1

Vaginal and Non-Vaginal Symptom Severity Scores for 25 Patients on Partial Treatment (weeks 0-32) and Full Treatment (weeks 32-58)

Symptom	Week 0 Mean	Week 0 SD	Week 32 Mean	Week 32 SD	Week 58 Mean	Week 58 SD	Difference 58-32	Confidence Interval	p<
Vaginal Pruritis	1.84	0.67	0.96	0.82	0.40	0.63	-0.56	-0.84 ↔ -0.27	0.005
Vaginal Burning	1.68	0.79	0.92	0.93	0.32	0.61	-0.60	-0.84 ↔ -0.35	0.0005
Vaginal Discharge	2.00	0.85	0.96	0.87	0.64	0.62	-0.32	-0.62 ↔ -0.01	0.05
VSS Mean	1.83	0.78	0.95	0.88	0.45	0.64	-0.49	-0.64 ↔ -0.33	0.0005
Abdominal Bloating	2.12	0.71	1.76	0.95	0.72	0.72	-1.04	-1.31 ↔ -0.76	0.0005
Abdominal Pain	1.56	0.80	1.28	0.92	0.36	0.48	-0.92	-1.19 ↔ -0.64	0.0005
Nausea	1.76	0.71	1.56	0.90	0.52	0.57	-1.04	-1.27 ↔ -0.80	0.0005
Diarrhea	0.64	0.79	0.16	0.37	0.08	0.27	-0.08	-0.21 ↔ 0.056	ns
Constipation	1.84	0.97	1.60	0.98	0.56	0.57	-1.04	-1.29 ↔ -0.78	0.0005
Perianal Pruritis	1.44	0.70	0.68	0.84	0.24	0.43	-0.44	-0.72 ↔ -0.15	0.01
Menstrual Irregularity	1.48	1.20	0.64	0.79	0.40	0.75	-0.24 *		0.01
Premenstrual Distress	2.60	0.89	1.92	1.13	0.84	0.92	-1.08	-1.42 ↔ -0.73	0.0005
Memory	2.04	0.77	1.84	0.92	0.76	0.65	-1.08	-1.35 ↔ -0.80	0.0005
Concentration	2.24	0.76	1.92	0.89	0.68	0.68	-1.24	-1.52 ↔ -0.95	0.0005
Depression	2.28	0.78	1.64	1.02	0.76	0.91	-0.88	-1.19 ↔ -0.56	0.0005
Lethargy	2.24	0.51	1.72	1.04	0.72	0.60	-1.00	-1.41 ↔ -0.58	0.0005
Rhinitis	2.20	1.10	1.88	1.21	0.92	0.89	-0.96	-1.36 ↔ -0.55	0.0005
Sneezing	0.72	0.72	0.60	0.69	0.20	0.40	-0.40	-0.62 ↔ -0.17	0.005
Wheezing	0.76	0.86	0.84	1.08	0.28	0.72	-0.56	-0.87 ↔ -0.24	0.005
NVSS Mean	1.73	1.03	1.34	1.10	0.54	0.71	-0.80	-0.87 ↔ -0.72	0.0005

-- Week 0 = pre-treatment; Week 32 = end of partial treatment (nystatin/placebo); Week 58 = end of full treatment (oral and vaginal nystatin and diet)

-- Severity of symptoms scored on a 0-3 scale. VSS mean = mean of vaginal symptom scores. NVSS mean = mean of non-vaginal symptom scores.

-- Confidence interval = 95% interval (mean difference, week 32-58 ± t.05 ´ standard error of difference)

-- p values determined by correlated t-test, one-tail, df = 24

* At Week 32, 14 of the 25 patients had no symptoms (score of 0), and eleven patients scored a 1 or 2. At Week 58, seven patients improved, one was worse, and three were unchanged. Improvement of these 11 patients was significant, p<.01, one-tail, by correlated t-test.

Table 2A

Pre- and Post-treatment GTT Results

	GTT time (minutes)	Group A (pretreatment only)				Group B (pretreatment)				Group C (post-treatment)				Group D (post-treatment only)			
		n	mean	St. Dev.	SEm	n	mean	St. Dev.	SEm	n	mean	St. Dev.	SEm	n	mean	St. Dev.	SEm
glucose (mg%)	0	44	80.98	9.60	1.45	9	80.89	9.56	3.19	9	77.00	8.11	2.70	13	84.46	9.44	2.62
glucose (mg%)	30	41	149.17	51.15	7.99	8	149.00	40.34	14.26	9	136.00	34.59	11.53	13	139.54	44.19	12.26
glucose (mg%)	60	43	132.28	54.28	8.28	9	161.67	47.60	15.87	9	125.67	37.72	12.57	13	117.77	38.87	10.78
glucose (mg%)	90	43	116.02	36.63	5.59	9	140.00	48.92	16.31	9	107.89	40.51	13.50	13	101.85	29.51	8.19
glucose (mg%)	120	43	96.07	27.96	4.26	9	126.67	49.32	16.44	9	99.22	30.52	10.17	13	89.42	22.00	6.35
insulin (μIU/mL)	0	37	18.19	9.52	1.57	9	24.78	23.44	7.81	9	15.11	9.37	3.12	13	16.85	5.46	1.51
insulin (μIU/mL)	30	34	132.03	62.93	10.79	8	120.00	85.41	30.20	9	85.89	45.54	15.18	12	96.50	70.96	20.48
insulin (μIU/mL)	60	34	176.44	103.64	17.77	8	196.88	100.40	35.50	9	94.11	40.50	13.50	12	106.92	75.52	21.80
insulin (μIU/mL)	90	36	175.00	107.55	17.92	9	196.56	154.77	51.59	9	95.44	61.41	20.47	11	74.73	46.29	13.96
insulin (μIU/mL)	120	36	127.33	93.25	15.54	9	171.33	186.95	62.32	9	93.78	62.44	20.81	11	69.82	73.74	22.23
FFA (mEq/L)	0	37	0.704	0.269	0.044	9	0.774	0.365	0.122	9	0.483	0.231	0.077	13	0.682	0.289	0.080
FFA (mEq/L)	30	34	0.299	0.128	0.022	6	0.459	0.211	0.086	9	0.221	0.130	0.043	12	0.276	0.102	0.029
FFA (mEq/L)	60	35	0.202	0.092	0.016	9	0.235	0.080	0.027	9	0.143	0.064	0.021	12	0.170	0.061	0.018
FFA (mEq/L)	90	35	0.148	0.076	0.013	9	0.181	0.081	0.027	9	0.094	0.038	0.013	11	0.125	0.070	0.021
FFA (mEq/L)	120	36	0.130	0.073	0.012	9	0.137	0.120	0.040	9	0.081	0.039	0.013	11	0.097	0.059	0.018

Group A consists of pretreatment GTT studies on 53 patients. Group B is a subgroup of Group A, comprised of 9 patients for whom post-treatment GTT's were available, and who followed the entire treatment protocol. Group C shows post-treatment studies on the 9 full treatment patients. Group D consists of 13 patients with the same symptoms and treatment as Group B/C, but who did not complete pretreatment GTT studies.

Table 2B

Pre- and Post-treatment GTT Results Comparison

	GTT time	A vs B				B vs C				A vs D				C vs D			
	(minutes)	mean diff	t	df	p< (2 tail)	mean diff	t	df	p< (1tail)	mean diff	t	df	p< (1tail)	mean diff	t	df	p< (2 tail)
glucose (mg%)	0	0.09	0.03	11.55	ns	3.89	1.33	8	ns	-3.48	-1.16	19.93	ns	-7.46	-1.98	18.94	ns
glucose (mg%)	30	0.17	0.01	11.88	ns	20.75	1.15	7	ns	9.63	0.66	23.11	ns	-3.54	-0.21	19.61	ns
glucose (mg%)	60	-29.39	-1.64	12.77	ns	36.00	2.09	8	0.05	14.51	1.07	27.58	ns	7.90	0.48	17.71	ns
glucose (mg%)	90	-23.98	-1.39	9.96	ns	32.11	1.96	8	0.05	14.17	1.43	24.28	ns	6.04	0.38	13.72	ns
glucose (mg%)	120	-30.60	-1.80	9.10	ns	27.44	1.47	8	ns	6.65	0.89	24.89	ns	9.80	0.83	13.62	ns
insulin (μIU/mL	0	-6.59	-0.83	8.65	ns	9.67	1.59	8	ns	1.34	0.62	37.18	ns	-1.74	-0.50	11.77	ns
insulin (μIU/mL	30	12.03	0.38	8.87	ns	32.50	1.39	7	ns	35.53	1.53	17.50	ns	-10.61	-0.42	18.66	ns
insulin (μIU/mL	60	-20.44	-0.51	10.81	ns	97.38	2.92	7	0.01	69.52	2.47	26.57	0.01	-12.81	-0.50	17.51	ns
insulin (μIU/mL	90	-21.56	-0.39	10.01	ns	101.11	2.02	8	0.05	100.27	4.41	39.49	0.00005	20.71	0.84	14.64	ns
insulin (μIU/mL	120	-44.00	-0.69	9.02	ns	77.56	1.26	8	ns	57.51	2.12	20.75	0.05	23.96	0.79	17.96	ns
FFA (mEq/L)	0	-0.07	-0.54	10.21	ns	0.29	1.74	8	ns	0.02	0.24	19.81	ns	-0.20	-1.79	19.48	ns
FFA (mEq/L)	30	-0.16	-1.80	5.67	ns	0.24	2.29	5	0.05	0.02	0.63	24.14	ns	-0.06	-1.05	14.80	ns
FFA (mEq/L)	60	-0.03	-1.07	13.99	ns	0.09	2.76	8	0.01	0.03	1.36	29.12	ns	-0.03	-0.98	16.91	ns
FFA (mEq/L)	90	-0.03	-1.10	11.89	ns	0.09	3.78	8	0.005	0.02	0.93	18.05	ns	-0.03	-1.26	15.92	ns
FFA (mEq/L)	120	-0.01	-0.17	9.53	ns	0.06	1.37	8	ns	0.03	1.53	20.28	ns	-0.02	-0.73	17.35	ns

ns = not significant

There are no significant differences between Group A and Group B; therefore their data, separate here, are combined (total n = 53) for pre-treatment comparisons with other groups.

There are no significant differences between Group C and Group D, showing Group D should reflect what might be expected of Group C after several years of treatment.

Changes with treatment were significant overall (by binomial theorem) since all changes were in the same direction.

APPENDIX I

Long-term Follow-up
Four Cases

A natural question that arises relates to the chance of recurrence among patients who were seriously ill before being restored to normal health by treatment that returned Candida albicans to its role as a relatively harmless member of the body's "normal flora."

A unique opportunity presented itself in several of the severe cases used in *The Missing Diagnosis* to illustrate the principles being reported. These are indeed "long-term" follow-ups consisting of up to 25 years since they were first presented. The details of each case may be found in *The Missing Diagnosis* on the pages indicated.

Case 1: (page 128—softcover) This 36-year-old woman, treated with drugs and many episodes of electric shock therapy for severe, long-standing schizophrenia, was scheduled for permanent commitment to the state mental hospital when she presented with symptoms of chronic yeast overgrowth that had begun with pregnancy at age 25 years. She was well 12 weeks after beginning yeast treatment.

Ten years later she walked into the office with a big smile on her face. She had moved to North Carolina and had "stopped by just to let me know she had been fine."

Case 4: (page 134—softcover) This is the case of the nurse, age 36 years, who almost died from 3 self-inflicted gunshot wounds to the chest. Eight weeks after beginning anti-yeast therapy she was so well that her psychiatrist dismissed her.

I continued to see her regularly for treatment of her hay fever. She continued to be in charge of a 300-bed nursing home until she retired. She remained completely well mentally. Significantly, there was never a recurrence of the many kidney stones that had occurred from age 25 until age 36. (This had also happened in the case of her father. See Case 5.)

Case 5: (page 136—softcover) This is the case of the man, age 60, who developed the intractable eye inflammation that had resisted all therapy, including antibiotics and steroids. (He was the father of the young woman described in Case 4.) This eye condition had cleared with anti-yeast treatment.

This man had been under the care of a urologist because of chronic urinary tract infections and kidney stones. Over a period of 20 years he had passed many stones, and stones had been removed from each kidney. As in the case of his daughter (Case 4), from beginning anti-yeast therapy he never developed another stone.

He lived and farmed for many years until his death from a stroke. Treatment had also cleared the severe lethargy that also had been present. He continued on nystatin because every effort to discontinue treatment led to return of the lethargy and constipation, although there was never a recurrence of the eye inflammation, which may well have been due to an autoimmune mechanism.

Chemical intolerance—Case 2: (page 57—softcover) This was the patient who at age 27 developed the severe reaction to chemical odors, e.g., perfumes, hairsprays, exhaust fumes, pesticides, cleaners, etc. Seen first at age 30 years, he had been totally impotent for 2 years. He made full recovery, and at age 59 years he is still racing and winning (for his age category). He has taken nystatin intermittently over the years because he tends to have some recurrence of bloating and constipation; however, there has been no recurrence of the severe chemical intolerance or impotence.

These few cases tell us what the future may hold for these few patients whose problem with Candida albicans became so severe. Nystatin continues to help with the Candida-induced symptoms usually diagnosed as "irritable bowel syndrome."

The father-daughter patients who experienced total relief from long-standing problems with kidney stones are intriguing and may point the way to further exploration into yeast as a cause of at least some varieties of kidney stones.

Finally, it has been most encouraging that there has been no recurrence of extremely severe cases of mental illness, eye inflammation, impotence, etc. We can feel safe in concluding that with reasonable attention to diet and to the overuse of antibiotics, steroids, and birth-control pills, Candida albicans will remain where it belongs.

It will be of *great* interest to see what future research uncovers as to the mechanisms by which the many (79) antigens coming from Candida albicans are disrupting human physiology—just how many as yet unrecognized problems with human health are yeast related.

Highly important is the lesson we are taught by Case 3 (page 133—softcover). This man had developed a puzzling skin lesion (biopsied 3 times) 7 years before his first visit, and severe asthma 5 years earlier. However, his bowel function was fine—totally asymptomatic—until 3 years earlier. Thus the "local" symptoms where the yeast had infected the colon were *entirely* absent for 4 years and 2 years respectively, during which developed the "generalized" symptoms in the skin and lungs. Had I seen him 3 years earlier, there would have been no colon symptoms to alert me to the *cause* of the tumor and asthma.

Thus, the numerous (79) substances (antigens) being fed into the body may *precede* any *local* symptoms arising at the site where the yeast has gained access to the bloodstream (the colon in *this* case). The conclusion to be drawn is that in virtually any condition in which the etiology (cause) is obscure, this mechanism is worth considering for a brief therapeutic trial of yeast suppression with nystatin and diet. Until such time as a definitive test of blood or urine becomes available, I see no alternative to such a brief therapeutic trial to see if any of a patient's symptoms are altered by thus interrupting the entry into the bloodstream of these many yeast products.

APPENDIX II

PREVIOUS PUBLICATIONS

The following papers are reprinted with the kind permission of the publishers,

the *Journal of Orthomolecular Psychiatry* and

the *Journal of Advancement in Medicine.*

REPRINTED FROM
The Journal of Orthomolecular Psychiatry
Volume 13 Number 2
Publication Office: 2229 Broad Street, Regina, Saskatchewan, Canada. Published Quarterly. Reproduction without permission is prohibited.

Metabolic Abnormalities in Patients with Chronic Candidiasis

The Acetaldehyde Hypothesis

C. Orian Truss, M.D.[1]

Introduction

Mold sensitivity is common among allergy patients, occurring alone or in association with reactions to foods and to other inhalants, such as house dust, animal danders, and the pollens of weeds, grasses, and trees.

Symptoms of allergy result from an altered reaction to substances encountered in the environment. Contact with food is primarily intestinal, while that with pollen and house dust is principally respiratory.

Mold exposure, however, is abundant by both routes. Mold spores are prevalent in inhaled air, especially in damp weather and in environments that are "musty". Patients commonly develop symptoms from hay, leaves, basement air, feather pillows, and house plants. In addition to these inhaled spores, much exposure occurs in the intestine from molds that are in or on foods; fruits, aged cheeses, breads and pastries, and vinegar and alcoholic beverages are prominent among the foods that have a high yeast content.

The most effective treatment of allergies is avoidance. When contact with the allergen can be minimized to a sufficient degree, other treatment is unnecessary. Allergies that may be completely controlled in this way include those to foods, drugs, animal dander, and poison ivy. When complete avoidance is not possible, minimizing exposure to the allergen aids greatly in controlling symptoms; better house dust control is an example.

Mold avoidance includes the elimination of house plants, wet basements and other sources of excess humidity, and foods with a high yeast content. This is an essential part of treatment. In fact, without this, results from the remainder of the treatment program often will be disappointing.

When contact cannot be reduced sufficiently to adequately control symptoms, standard allergy treatment includes the injection of extracts of the allergen, usually over an extended period. Often called "hyposensitization," this may effectively control symptoms that remain despite maximum avoidance. Such extracts are used in treating pollen, house dust, and mold allergies, since contact is inevitable with these allergens that are in the air we must breathe, and often only minimal benefit is realized from the use of antihistamines. Some think that this therapy relieves the symptoms of allergy by

[1]. 2614 Highland Ave., Birmingham, Alabama 35205
Presented at the Yeast-Human Interaction Conference, December 10, 1983, Birmingham, Alabama.

stimulating the formation of IgG or "blocking" antibodies, or perhaps by an effect on suppressor T-cells.

Thus, to summarize, total avoidance of the allergen is the perfect and only treatment necessary, as for food allergies. When this is not possible, as with allergens in the air, immunotherapy with extracts of the allergens is used to alleviate symptoms. The principle of trying to control immunologically those symptoms that cannot be eliminated by avoidance is common to the methods of most allergists, although there may be differences in their methods of administering the extracts.

The purpose of this brief discussion has been to consider the principles that apply to allergy treatment in general, so that we might point out a third element that is uniquely characteristic of mold sensitivity.

In addition to mold allergens that are derived from air and food, others are produced by fungi living on the surface-coverings of the human body. Skin and mucous membranes normally are colonized by living organisms that are the source of antigens to which we may become allergic. When these organisms are fungi, mold allergens actively produced in the body are added to the mold in food and in inhaled air, and quantitatively may be of great importance in the total mold load.

Since the amount of fungus colonizing tissues will have much to do with its contribution to the total mold load, an important addition to treatment will be made by measures that reduce the growth of mold in the mucous membranes and skin.

The "id" reaction to trichophyton was perhaps the first reported example of an allergic response distant from the site of growth of the fungus producing the allergen. However, of the various fungi living in the human body, Candida albicans is quantitatively the most important, since it colonizes the entire intestinal tract and vagina, lives on skin, and may infect nails. Patients with mold sensitivity often describe great difficulty in controlling "athlete's foot," as well as fungous infections of the nails, vagina, and intestines. Frequently these cease to be a problem with successful therapy of the patients' mold sensitivity. Allergenic extracts of trichophyton, Candida albicans, aspergillus, and other fungi that so colonize the human body are used widely in the treatment of mold sensitivity. They are used singly or as part of mixtures of mold allergens. One particular combination used widely is TOE, containing extracts of Trichophyton, Candida albicans, and Epidermophyton.

A second reason that Candida albicans has become of great importance in this clinical problem is that its growth is strongly stimulated by antibiotics, contraceptive hormones, and immunosuppressant drugs. For the past 35 years the increasing use of these substances in medical practice has adversely affected the growth of this yeast in many individuals. It has become a major factor in mold sensitivity, and indeed, in many cases may eventually become the predominant problem.

In the overall treatment program for mold sensitivity, measures of avoidance should include an attempt to minimize the impact of these factors that increase the growth of this yeast in the human body. This includes greater care in determining the indication for the use of antibiotics and steroid hormones, and the selection of alternate methods of birth control in patients with mold sensitivity.

Yeast growth may also be suppressed by the use of standard anti-fungal medication. Several are available, nystatin being the most widely used. It has been used for over 30 years to treat "thrush" in infants, vaginitis in women and girls, and intestinal symptoms due to yeast in both sexes and at all ages. Finally, we may add standard Candida albicans extract to those of the other molds used in immunotherapy.

Although Candida albicans cannot be avoided completely, its contribution to the total mold exposure can be minimized by thus applying to it the principles of avoidance and immunotherapy common to the treatment of other allergies.

Treatment of the chronic yeast infection, besides contributing to the overall control of mold sensitivity, is important in itself. This infection may become so severe that it dominates the clinical picture. The original symptoms of inhalant mold allergy may have become less important than those of the "chronic candidiasis" that has evolved as a result of the yeast susceptibility that is part of the problem of mold sensitivity.

The contribution of this fungus to the total clinical picture in patients susceptible to its overgrowth led to the metabolic studies presented in this paper. Clinical observations on this subject were first presented in 1977 (Truss, 1977). Three subsequent papers (Truss, 1978; 1980; 1981) and a book (Truss, 1983) about illness caused by this yeast described its manifestations, the factors that precipitate and aggravate it, and its treatment.

It was stressed throughout that, because of its universal presence in the human body, commonly used diagnostic techniques reveal little about this condition, and that the diagnosis must be suspected from the clinical picture and confirmed by the response to treatment of its various manifestations.

Because of the desirability of establishing a laboratory basis for the diagnosis of this condition, studies were initiated in 24 patients considered classic cases of mold sensitivity and chronic yeast susceptibility. Patients with this condition usually exhibit symptoms that are severe and of long duration. It seemed likely that such symptoms reflect underlying disturbances in basic metabolic pathways. If so, laboratory evidence of such disturbances would aid both in the diagnosis of this condition, and in the assessment of its status during treatment.

The design of this study was to carry out a general evaluation of protein, fat, and carbohydrate metabolism, with the addition of more specific studies later if indicated by abnormalities brought out in the study's initial phase. Accordingly, pre-treatment determinations included amino acids in the urine, fatty acids in plasma and erythrocyte membranes, and intermediates of the glycolytic pathway.

In addition, special studies were incorporated to test the hypothesis that acetaldehyde, produced in the intestine by the anaerobic fermentation of sugars by Candida albicans, is the principal mediator of metabolic disturbances surfacing clinically as the symptoms of this condition.

Reported in this paper are the results of measurements before treatment in 24 patients, together with results in seven of the 24 who were restudied after varying periods of treatment, and following substantial clinical improvement. The toxicity of acetaldehyde is reviewed, and the hypothesis presented that this substance is the major toxin responsible for the metabolic abnormalities found in these patients. The concluding discussion considers the laboratory findings in these patients in terms of acetaldehyde toxicity, and presents facts pertinent to the concept that fermentation of sugars by Candida albicans underlies the physiologic disturbances manifested by the many symptoms characteristic of this condition.

The Acetaldehyde Hypothesis

Patients with an overgrowth of yeast in the intestine exhibit much gas formation following the ingestion of sugar or digestible carbohydrates. This is evidenced clinically by abdominal distention, excess flatus, and belching. The metabolism of sugar by yeasts releases carbon dioxide (CO_2), whether this be under anaerobic (fermentation) or aerobic conditions.

Formation of Acetaldehyde in Vitro

In yeasts, pyruvate is produced from sugar by glycolysis, just as in human cells. If oxygen is not available, many species of yeast decarboxylate the pyruvate to acetaldehyde, which is then reduced to ethanol. If oxygen is present, pyruvate is oxidatively decarboxylated to acetyl Co-enzyme A (acetyl CoA), and acetaldehyde and ethanol are not formed. Therefore, in many types of yeast the fate of pyruvate (and therefore of sugar) is determined primarily by the availability, or lack thereof, of oxygen. Most strains of Candida albicans, however, are not able to convert acetaldehyde to ethanol to any significant degree, but can under anaerobic conditions convert pyruvate to acetaldehyde. We will return later to the potential significance of this in the human body.

Yeasts also are able to metabolize ethanol to acetaldehyde, if oxygen is available. The ethanol may be supplied exogenously, or produced by the yeast itself. Thus ethanol that has resulted from anaerobic fermentation will be quickly oxidized to acetaldehyde as soon as oxygen is available.

Candida albicans is one species of yeast that is able to accomplish in vitro this conversion of ethanol to acetaldehyde when oxygen is available. (If it can do so also in the intestine, this pathway would provide an additional source of acetaldehyde, since small amounts of ethanol are produced normally by intestinal bacteria.)

Thus there are two pathways for the generation of acetaldehyde by Candida albicans: (1) the conversion of pyruvate to acetaldehyde when oxygen is not available and (2) the conversion of ethanol (exogenous or endogenous) to acetaldehyde when oxygen is available.

It is possible that most strains of Candida albicans produce ethanol in the human intestine, but in an amount too small to be detectable in the peripheral blood. That the intestinal environment is sufficiently anaerobic for this to occur is indicated by the fact that, if adequate sugar is available, certain strains of Candida albicans can produce ethanol in quantities sufficient to induce a rising blood-alcohol level, and clinical drunkenness (Iwata, 1972). Thus such strains can efficiently accomplish the final step in ethanol production, i.e., the conversion of acetaldehyde to ethyl alcohol. Therefore, these special strains of Candida albicans are capable of accomplishing in the human intestine the two reactions by which pyruvate is anaerobically converted to ethanol:

(1) Pyruvate + $H^+ \longrightarrow$ acetaldehyde + CO_2

(2) Acetaldehyde + NADH + $H^+ \longrightarrow$ ethanol + NAD^+

Common strains of Candida albicans, although largely incapable of accomplishing reaction (2), are able under anaerobic conditions in vitro to convert pyruvate to acetaldehyde and CO_2. The production of ethanol is minimal or absent (Van Niel and Anderson, 1941; Van Niel and Cohen, 1942).

If the same reactions prevail in vivo, the large amount of gas generated in the intestinal tract when patients with yeast overgrowth eat carbohydrate would be the CO_2 liberated by the decarboxylation of pyruvate, as shown in equation (1). Acetaldehyde would be the remaining product.

Fate of Acetaldehyde

The major mechanism for the disposition of aldehydes in the body is oxidation by means of aldehyde dehydrogenase. This takes place primarily in the liver, although other tissues to some extent aid in this process. When the aldehyde is acetaldehyde, the oxidation product is acetate, which binds to Co-enzyme A (CoA). The acetyl CoA so formed may undergo any of the normal fates of acetyl CoA. Thus the acetyl group may condense with oxaloacetate for oxidation in the citric acid cycle; it may be utilized for the synthesis of ketones, cholesterol, and fatty acids; or it may be donated by acetyl CoA for the synthesis of acetylcholine and other compounds requiring this two-carbon molecule.

Because of the efficiency of aldehyde oxidation, this toxin accumulates in the bloodstream only when its formation is excessively great and prolonged. Acetaldehyde is the first oxidation product of ethanol, yet may remain undetectable in the blood when alcohol consumption is moderate. Its accumulation in the blood occurs only if the rate of alcohol consumption is sufficient to saturate the acetaldehyde oxidizing mechanism.

The importance of this observation is not so much that the acetaldehyde oxidizing mechanism can finally be saturated, but rather that the production of a large amount of acetaldehyde can occur without its being detectable in the bloodstream. A high blood level of alcohol may co-exist with a normal blood level of acetaldehyde, and yet the eventual disappearance of alcohol from the blood means that acetaldehyde has been generated at a rate comparable to the rate of alcohol oxidation.

Although oxidation accounts for the removal from the bloodstream of most acetaldehyde, a second mechanism may be responsible for the disappearance of a significant amount. A strong affinity exists between acetaldehyde and tissues. This rests at least in part on its ability to bind to sulfhydryl and amine groups. Such binding delays the accumulation in the blood of this toxin, and also protects it from oxidation by aldehyde dehydrogenase.

It is not possible to estimate the amount of acetaldehyde that might remain intact because of such protective binding. This mechanism may account for only a small portion of the acetaldehyde removed from the blood, although its contribution relative to oxidation may vary with the rate of acetaldehyde production. Once the rate of its formation exceeds the oxidizing capacity of the liver, it will appear in the peripheral blood, making possible its binding to tissues throughout the body. It seems likely, also, that its binding to amine and sulfhydryl groups will be cumulative when it is generated chronically, even though in small amount.

Formation of Acetaldehyde in Vivo by Candida Albicans

If, as proposed in this hypothesis, Candida albicans is capable of fermenting sugars to acetaldehyde in the human intestine, the amount formed should be influenced by the following:

1. The availability of sugar for conversion into pyruvate by glycolysis.
2. The degree of anaerobiasis.
3. The quantity of viable yeast cells in the intestine, and their fermenting efficiency.
4. Other intestinal environmental factors that might be capable of influencing glycolysis or fermentation by Candida albicans, e.g., pH, bacterial flora.

Fate of Acetaldehyde Formed in Vivo by Candida Albicans

Acetaldehyde formed in this way would enter the portal circulation and, in the liver, undergo oxidization to acetate. It is unlikely that a quantity of acetaldehyde sufficient to saturate liver aldehyde dehydrogenase would be generated by most strains of Candida albicans. (That it could occur, however, is suggested by experience with the ethanol-producing strains.) Therefore, it would be unlikely that acetaldehyde formation in the intestine could be detected by measurement of its level in the peripheral blood.

Thus, in this situation, opportunity for acetaldehyde to bind to sulfhydryl and amine groups would be limited to the time between its formation in the intestine and its oxidation in the liver. Although brief, this interval would allow contact with enzymes, and with constituents of the intestinal wall, liver cells, and portal blood. The latter would include nutrients as well as serum proteins, the latter having been found to bind acetaldehyde. Also exposed to acetaldehyde in the portal blood would be platelets, leukocytes, and erythrocytes. The release of acetaldehyde from erythrocytes was reported in 1941 (Barker, 1941).

Therefore, the presence of acetaldehyde in the intestine, the intestinal wall, and in the portal blood would afford many opportunities for its binding to such substances as nutrients, enzymes, vitamins, and polypeptides. If formed high in the intestinal tract, acetaldehyde could react with digestive enzymes in the small intestine. The possiblities are many.

Although the time available for binding is brief, presumably the same erythrocytes, leukocytes, and serum proteins come around repeatedly, each passage through the portal vessels exposing them to the cumulative effect of newly formed acetaldehyde, just as would occur in the fixed cells of the intestinal wall and liver. The ultimate effect of this very toxic substance could include disruption of intestinal absorptive processes, as well as impairment of function in erythrocytes, leukocytes, and other cells in which it accumulates.

As we will see in the next section, the known toxic effects of acetaldehyde are more than adequate to account for the metabolic disturbances found in the patients who were the subjects of this study. We know that common strains of Candida albicans produce acetaldehyde when they ferment sugars anaerobically in vitro. That they can do so in the human body remains to be demonstrated.

Toxicity of Acetaldehyde

Because acetaldehyde is produced by the intial step in the oxidation of ethyl alcohol, its toxic effects have received much attention in studies of alcohol addiction and toxicity. Many of the metabolic disturbances caused by acetaldehyde have been attributed to its strong affinity for sulfhydryl (-SH) and amine groups, and to the increase in the ratio of NADH to NAD that results from the oxidation of acetaldehyde by aldehyde dehydrogenase. This discussion will focus on the physiologic consequences of such acetaldehyde binding and oxidation.

Schiff Base Formation

The condensation of an aldehyde and an amine results in the formation of a Schiff base. An example of Schiff base formation in normal metabolism is the reaction of pyridoxal phosphate (PLP) with the amine group of an amino acid, as this co-enzyme participates in transamination reactions.

PLP is normally protected from degradation by its binding to the amine group of lysine residues of proteins, including serum proteins and hemoglobin. Acetaldehyde may, by binding preferentially to these residues, displace PLP and result in its increased destruction, and in abnormally low blood levels of this co-enzyme (Lumeng and Ting-Kai Li, 1974; Veitch et al., 1975).

Acetaldehyde may also bind to the amine group of neurotransmitters to form complex compounds that may function as "false neurotransmitters" (Cohen and Collins, 1970; Davis and Walsh, 1970). These have been demonstrated in minute amount in human urine (Sandler et al., 1973). It has been proposed that these substances are related in some way to alcohol addiction. Little is known about their effect on normal physiology, but it might be anticipated that it would depend upon the particular neurotransmitter involved in the condensation with acetaldehyde, just as does the name of the condensation product. For example, the tetrahydroisoquinoline that results from the condensation of dopamine and acetaldehyde is salsolinol. Condensation of acetaldehyde with indolealkylamines leads to the formation of tetrahydro-B-carbolines.

Other opportunities for Schiff-base formation undoubtedly exist where amine groups are available to participate in this reaction with acetaldehyde. The examples cited illustrate two areas of physiology that could be profoundly affected by this mechanism.

Sulfhydryl Binding

Aldehydes react with sulfhydryl groups to form hemiacetals. The -SH group is active in many metabolic steps. For example, it is involved in the first oxidative step of glycolysis, being essential to the activity of glyceraldehyde dehydrogenase, the enzyme that catalyzes the conversion of glyceraldehyde 3-phosphate to 1,3 diphosphoglycerate. The sulfhydryl group is also the active site of Coenzyme A (CoA). It is the -SH site of CoA that binds the acetyl group to form acetyl CoA.

CoA serves as carrier of the acetyl groups that are derived from carbohydrates, fats, and certain amino acids. Thus acetyl CoA is the point of convergence in the metabolism of the three classes of food, for their subsequent entry into and further oxidation by the citric acid cycle. Acetyl CoA also provides the two carbon units from which are synthesized fatty acids, ketones, and cholesterol and steroid hormones, and it donates the acetyl group required for the synthesis of acetylcholine and other substances.

There is possibly no single point in metabolic pathways more pivotal than acetyl CoA, nor one at which interference would have more far-reaching consequences in all organs of the body.

Ammon has shown in both brain and liver homogenates that acetaldehyde induces a dose-dependent suppression of acetyl CoA activity (Ammon et al., 1969; Ammon et al., 1971). He further showed that this was due to blocking of the active -SH group of CoA, which he believed to be due to the binding of acetaldehyde at this site. Finally, he demonstrated decreased respiration in these tissues, oxygen consumption falling in parallel with the declining level of acetyl CoA as the concentration of acetaldehyde increased.

Glyceraldehyde dehydrogenase and acetyl CoA are two examples of sites at which the integrity of -SH groups is essential in normal metabolic pathways. As is true for amine groups and Schiff-base formation, sulfhydryl groups are important at many additional sites in metabolic pathways, each offering the opportunity for acetaldehyde to exert its toxic effect by this mechanism.

Redox Potential

When the ratio of NADH/NAD increases, many secondary abnormalities occur. An uninterrupted supply of NAD is necessary in many areas of metabolism. NAD is converted to NADH when this nucleotide serves as hydrogen receptor in glycolysis, in the citric acid cycle, and elsewhere in metabolic reactions.

The amount of NAD in the body is quite limited. It is therefore imperative that it be regenerated continually for these processes to continue. Normally, by means of oxidative phosphorylation and the electron-transport chain, molecular oxygen eventually accepts the hydrogen from NADH, yielding ATP and NAD. The latter thus is again available for pathways that utilize it, such as glycolysis and the citric acid cycle.

When either ethanol or acetaldehyde is oxidized by its respective dehydrogenase, NAD is converted to NADH. When the necessity exists for the removal of these toxins in large amount over an extended period of time, the resulting shift to NADH decreases the amount of available NAD. The many metabolic transformations that utilize NAD as hydrogen receptor cannot proceed normally under these conditions.

An increased NADH/NAD ratio leads to many metabolic abnormalities. Some of the more important are listed. Lieber has recently reviewed the biochemical abnormalities that may occur in this situation (Lieber, 1980).

1. Increase in the ratio of lactate to pyruvate.
2. Increase in the ratio of plasma hydroxysteroids to ketosteroids.
3. Decreased galactose tolerance. The conversion of galactose to glucose is inhibited by NADH.
4. Alterations in amine metabolism. Where alternate pathways exist, reduced metabolites may be excreted at the expense of oxidized metabolites. One example is the altered metabolism of serotonin. The 5-HIAA (oxidative) pathway is inhibited by NADH. An increase in the reductive pathway results in the formation of more tryptophol. Thus the tryptophol /5-HIAA ratio is increased when NADH is present in excess relative to NAD.
5. The citric acid cycle is inhibited by NADH. Among the effects are:
    a.) Inhibition of fatty acid oxidation, which necessitates the disposal of excess fatty acids by a second mechanism involving ketone-body formation, and lipoprotein synthesis. Elevation of the B-hydroxybutyrate/acetoacetate ratio results from a high NADH/NAD ratio.
    b.) Inhibition of gluconeogenesis. Citric acid cycle intermediates are the entry points of many amino acids for their subsequent conversion to glycogen. Simultaneous inhibition of glycolysis by NADH, leading to decreased pyruvate production, increases the deficit of the citric acid cycle intermediate, oxaloacetate, with alteration of the malate/oxaloacetate ratio.
6. Inhibition of glycolysis by NADH at the first oxidative step (conversion of glyceraldehyde 3-PO_4 to 1,3 diphosphoglycerate). This inhibits energy release (ATP formation) as well as pyruvate formation. The deficiency of pyruvate reduces available oxaloacetate (derived from pyruvate) with which acetyl CoA must condense for acetate to enter the citric acid cycle.
7. Elevation of blood uric acid secondary to the elevated lactate levels caused by NADH excess. Lactate and uric acid compete for excretion in the kidney tubule.
8. Abnormalities in porphyrin metabolism. NAD is used in the conversion of coproporphyrin to protoporphyrin. Excess excretion of coproporphyrin results.
9. Oxidative phosphorylation is inhibited by acetaldehyde. This is reversed by NAD.
10. Decreased protein synthesis and increased proteolysis.

In addition to the effects of the high NADH/NAD ratio, Lieber lists the following toxic effects of acetaldehyde:

1. Reduction in the number of microtubules in the liver.
2. Decreased protein secretion, with protein retention in the liver.
3. Engorgement of the Golgi apparatus with VLDL particles.
4. Accumulation of lipid and protein, causing increased size of hepatocytes.
5. Depression of glutathione in the liver, possibly as a result of the binding of acetaldehyde to its cysteine component. Glutathione is important in the removal of toxic free-radicals; a reduction in glutathione may damage membranes. Lipid peroxidation and decreased GSH (reduced glutathione) occurred in animals following chronic ethanol intake.
6. Stimulation of hepatic smooth endoplasmic reticulum, leading to an increase in the rate of metabolism of alcohol and of drugs and, less desirably, to an increased rate of conversion of various substances to more toxic compounds.
7. The mitochondrial ethanol oxidizing system (MEOS) produces acetaldehyde in the endoplasmic reticulum, in contrast to that produced by alcohol dehydrogenase in the cytosol. This leads to greater acetaldehyde concentration at this site (i.e., endoplasmic reticulum), possibly with induction of enzymes that are important in carcinogenesis and in lipid peroxidation.
8. Increased collagen deposition in the liver (detectable only chemically in its early

stages, but later by light microscopy). This is thought to be due in part to the increased lactate associated with the high NADH/NAD ratio. This leads to an increase in peptidyl proline hydroxylase activity, favoring collagen deposition in other tissues as well as in the liver.

This brief summary lists only some of the suspected toxic effects of acetaldehyde. It indicates the profound and varied effects to be expected from prolonged exposure to this substance. The excellent review by Lieber provides a more detailed discussion of this subject, as well as a valuable bibliography of many of the papers pertaining to the metabolism of alcohol and acetaldehyde, and their effects in animals and humans.

Metabolic Studies in Patients With Chronic Candidiasis

Twenty-four patients with symptoms typical of mold sensitivity and yeast susceptibility were the subjects of a study designed to demonstrate, if possible, interference in pathways involved in the metabolism of proteins, fats, and carbohydrates. If present, abnormalities in the levels of enzymes, co-factors, or metabolic intermediates should be helpful in diagnosing this condition and, more importantly, in fostering an understanding of the patho-physiologic mechanisms that account for symptoms that bridge anatomical boundaries between different organ systems of the body. Findings to date in this continuing study are presented in this paper.

Additional studies have been selected specifically to test the hypothesis that acetaldehyde produced chronically in the body by Candida albicans is exerting significant toxic effects in these patients. The results of one of these studies are also presented.

In the initial screening studies, protein metabolism was evaluated by measurement of the 24-hour excretion of amino acids in the urine (Beckman 119 Amino Acid Analyzer). Specimens were collected the second 24 hours of a 48-hour period during which the patients were on low-protein diets.

Fat metabolism was evaluated by measuring fatty acids in plasma and in erythrocyte membranes. We are indebted to Dr. David Horrobin for these determinations.

Erythrocyte filtration was incorporated into the design of the study because acetaldehyde is known to cause increased rigidity of Rbc membranes, (Gaines, 1977; Palmer and Betts, 1975; Vassar et al., 1972) and because acetaldehyde has been demonstrated in red blood cells. (Barker, 1941).

In addition to the pre-treatment results in these twenty-four patients, repeat studies are presented in several following significant clinical improvement, the periods of treatment ranging from two to nine months. Special emphasis in the interpretation of all abnormalities is given to areas of metabolism thought to be affected by acetaldehyde.

24-Hour Amino-Acid Analyses

Of the 41 amino acids analyzed by the Beckman Amino Acid Analyzer, normal ranges have been established for 25 (Bio-Science Laboratories - Los Angeles, CA). In these 24 patients, many values outside the normal range were present before treatment (Table I). For certain important amino acids the abnormalities were severe, and were present either in all, or in a high percentage of these patients.

Caution is needed in interpreting the results of 24-hour amino acid excretion. This test is useful for the most part as a general evaluation of protein metabolism. Diet, of course, has a profound effect on the level of excretion of the essential amino acids. Also, it is probable that the normal ranges given will require modification as knowledge increases of these levels in healthy subjects.

Table II shows for each amino acid the percentage of these 24 patients with values that were normal, low, or elevated. For several amino acids exhibiting marked abnormality, bar graphs are used to show the values for each patient in relation to the normal range. The following trends may be seen in these findings:

1. Although occasional elevations are seen, the general tendency is one of values lower than normal.
2. Strikingly low are certain non-essential amino acids that derive their carbon skeletons from intermediates in the citric acid cycle:
   a.) glutamate (Figure 1) and glutamine (Figure 2), from alpha ketoglutarate
   b.) asparagine (Figure 3), from oxaloacetate
3. Relatively normal levels are present of non-essential amino acids derived from inter-

Table I

24-Hour Urine Amino Acid Determinations*

Amino Acids	Normal Values	Patients Before Treatment																							
		N.J.	L.G.	K.H.	J.C.	S.H.	A.G.	H.W.	J.W.	V.G.	J.H.	C.G.	J.P.	M.P.	M.S.	F.S.	E.M.	S.V.	S.B.	C.B.	K.W.	E.G.	J.B.	J.N.	R.B.
Taurine	63-2300	**7**	703	152	282	277	282	605	726	135	1042	200	391	281	**15**	1042	458	656	171	**7**	258	161	389	113	228
Phosphoethanolamine	26-101	**TR**	**TR**	**TR**	**TR**	**AB**	**TR**	**TR**	100	34	**TR**	**TR**	80	**TR**	**TR**	100	**TR**	97	**TR**	**21**	**TR**	**8**	42	**TR**	30
Aspartic	23-218	39	80	*220*	123	119	207	68	130	72	131	132	65	132	**39**	101	45	188	88	64	66	68	76	44	142
Threonine	85-440	**27**	**46**	120	**75**	**42**	**65**	**58**	**71**	102	**66**	**60**	**30**	237	**53**	**56**	**23**	104	**34**	**54**	**49**	**53**	88	**36**	142
Serine	160-700	**112**	**135**	649	163	**139**	246	**140**	192	316	242	**117**	**154**	885	**146**	191	**86**	330	164	**122**	193	**142**	224	**129**	294
Asparagine	270-700	**TR**	**23**	**TR**	**7**	**93**	**50**	**29**	**60**	**60**	**31**	**28**	**64**	**105**	**14**	**49**	**33**	**45**	**3**	**33**	**25**	**30**	**67**	**28**	**67**
Glutamic Acid	55-270	**TR**	94	**23**	**37**	**39**	**20**	**14**	**16**	**4**	**22**	**12**	**16**	**27**	**10**	**18**	**29**	**42**	**7**	**51**	**32**	**3**	**17**	**6**	**8**
a-aminoadipic Acid	31-81	**AB**	**TR**	**TR**	**16**	**9**	**TR**	**10**	**8**	36	**21**	**14**	**TR**	**10**	**TR**	**17**	**TR**	**TR**	**18**	**TR**	**8**	**22**	**17**	**AB**	32
Glycine	160-4200	567	467	3231	1210	1038	1200	628	872	3964	757	1041	839	*8683*	804	1466	391	2291	262	324	518	424	1291	551	992
Glutamine	140-860	**82**	**33**	476	**126**	**103**	161	**107**	**122**	180	**123**	**130**	**92**	650	**126**	230	**56**	282	**69**	148	**133**	**131**	244	**85**	320
Alanine	60-800	130	120	657	184	83	96	113	255	627	84	177	**57**	*802*	113	106	130	347	**37**	155	173	85	150	127	249
a-amino n-butyric	16-77	**TR**	21	28	**13**	**TR**	21	**8**	19	29	18	16	**8**	69	18	26	**TR**	38	**13**	**12**	22	16	34	**11**	32
Valine	14-51	**TR**	**TR**	30	**13**	**TR**	18	**TR**	22	27	**9**	18	**TR**	31	14	28	**TR**	16	**9**	**TR**	**11**	14	25	**TR**	31
Cystine	20-130	44	107	*131*	50	55	115	91	83	*174*	83	66	37	*255*	56	79	38	*138*	37	47	60	66	60	47	97
Methionine	20-95	**TR**	**TR**	**TR**	**13**	**14**	31	**18**	**16**	40	**19**	**12**	**13**	38	**14**	21	**12**	29	**12**	**10**	**14**	25	**14**	**13**	22
Cystathionine	16-63	**TR**	**TR**	**TR**	**TR**	**TR**	**TR**	**TR**	16	49	**TR**	**TR**	**7**	**TR**	**TR**	**15**	**TR**	**12**	**TR**	**TR**	**TR**	**7**	**TR**	**TR**	**12**
Isoleucine	18-210	**TR**	**TR**	58	**6**	**TR**	**8**	**TR**	**15**	**17**	29	**14**	**4**	**TR**	**4**	36	**TR**	**10**	**TR**	**3**	28	**6**	22	**TR**	**6**
Leucine	21-200	**TR**	**6**	51	**14**	22	**19**	**12**	**26**	26	34	**20**	**7**	26	**12**	39	**7**	26	**10**	**10**	25	**16**	25	**8**	23
Tyrosine	40-270	**15**	**27**	80	**33**	**22**	45	**31**	67	82	59	58	**17**	128	41	62	**12**	65	**12**	**32**	**34**	**31**	63	**27**	135
Phenylalanine	24-190	31	109	65	27	**21**	32	**20**	67	**20**	**18**	28	105	*228*	36	55	**10**	*218*	**17**	*258*	25	**15**	74	**16**	68
Ethanolamine	59-307	93	263	*367*	219	236	*724*	*398*	139	*325*	*380*	295	105	*438*	285	*450*	**43**	*492*	285	*324*	218	148	226	233	*453*
Lysine	48-640	**30**	118	85	**37**	**28**	153	102	119	*1407*	84	50	**19**	589	84	101	**26**	121	**36**	52	**46**	102	95	**34**	102
1-methylhistidine	130-930	**51**	**23**	**TR**	**13**	365	**80**	**118**	**54**	**TR**	**28**	**33**	**16**	425	**26**	171	**34**	**54**	279	**45**	**24**	*1010*	**46**	**21**	**38**
Histidine	130-2100	**119**	255	1019	290	173	266	312	688	1129	337	227	**97**	1164	314	671	**90**	417	**116**	261	236	236	545	197	730
3-methylhistidine	56-249	59	106	210	135	124	*267*	123	226	87	186	174	104	*333*	124	198	101	*281*	173	123	143	138	163	87	*312*

Shows the value of each amino acid in these 24 patients.
Depressed values are shown in boldface and elevated values are shown underlined in italics.
All values expressed in MCM/24 hours.

*** TR denotes trace**
AB denotes absent

METABOLIC ABNORMALITIES

24 Hour Urine Amino Acid Analysis

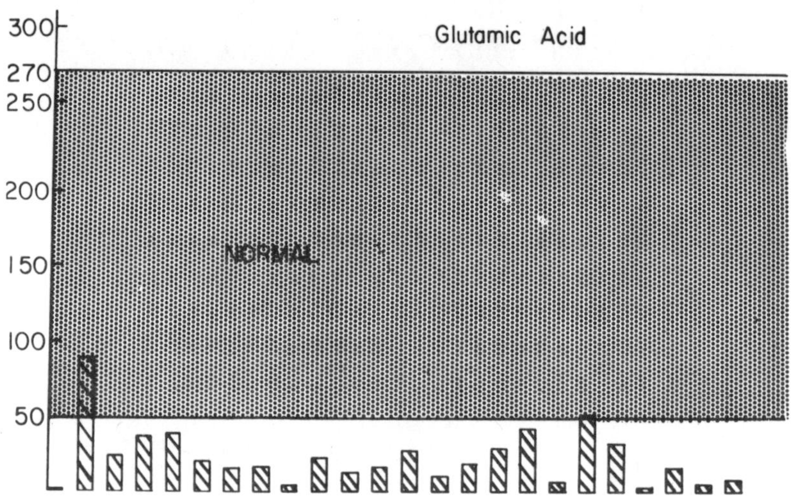

Glutamic acid excretion expressed in micromoles per 24 hours in 24 patients with chronic candidiasis.

mediates of the glycolytic pathway:

a.) alanine (from pyruvate)

b.) glycine (from 3 phosphoglycerate)

4. Ethanolamine levels generally are elevated, while those for phosphoethanolamine tend to be low. Since ethanolamine normally is converted to phosphoethanolamine, these results suggest a block in this pathway.

Taken as a whole, these findings suggest impairment in the synthesis of non-essential amino acids, particularly those synthesized from citric acid cycle intermediates. Such interconversions as ethanolamine to phosphoethanolamine, and aspartate to asparagine, appear inhibited. Attention is called to the very low levels of glutamate and glutamine, the donors of amine groups in transamination reactions.

Fatty Acid Levels in Plasma and in Erythrocyte Membranes

Plasma: Table III shows for these 24 patients the average levels of fatty acids of both the omega six and omega three series, together with the normal value for each fatty acid. The p values for the abnormalities found are shown.

Rbc membranes: Table IV shows similar studies and comparisons for fatty acids in the membranes of erythrocytes, with p values.

This same data is depicted graphically in Figure 4, which shows for each fatty acid in plasma and in Rbc membranes, the percent above or below normal of the average of the individual values before treatment. It will be noted that abnormalities were consistent throughout. In the omega six series the levels of the shorter chain fatty acids were elevated, while the levels of the longer chain fatty acids into which these are normally converted were depressed. Particularly striking were the very low levels of 22:5 omega six fatty acids.

Erythrocyte Filtration

The diameter of the human Rbc is approximately seven microns. These cells pass through capillaries of much smaller diameter,

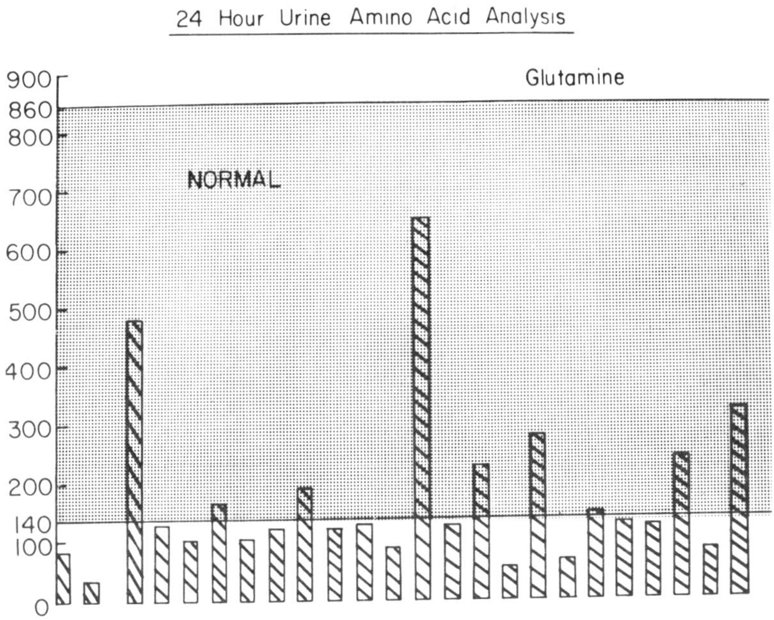

Figure 2:
Glutamine excretion expressed in micromoles per 24 hours in 24 patients with chronic candidiasis.

usually about two microns. In the sinusoids of the spleen, openings as small as one micron must be traversed. Maintenance of normal Rbc deformability is essential for these cells to accommodate to the small openings through which they must pass. Their ability to do so decreases as the rigidity of the Rbc membrane increases.

To estimate their flexibility in these patients, Rbc were filtered for one minute through filters three microns in diameter, with an applied vacuum of 20 cm water. To eliminate chance error due to a faulty filter, triplicate determinations were carried out, each with a new filter. The results were averaged and expressed as percent filtered in one minute. There was little variation in the three values, but when this occurred, the inconsistent result was disregarded and replaced with the result of a fourth filtration. Because this test was added later in the study, results are available for only eight of the 24 patients.

Figure 5 shows the results before and after treatment in these eight patients, together with results in eight healthy controls. The initial impairment of filtration is apparent, as is the striking improvement after treatment.

Post-Treatment Results

In addition to these eight filtration determinations, repeat measurements were obtained of 24-hour urinary amino acid excretion in seven patients, and of fatty acid levels in five patients. The intervals of treatment at the time of re-evaluation ranged from two to nine months.

24-hour Amino-Acid Levels in Urine

Figures 6 and 7 show graphically the

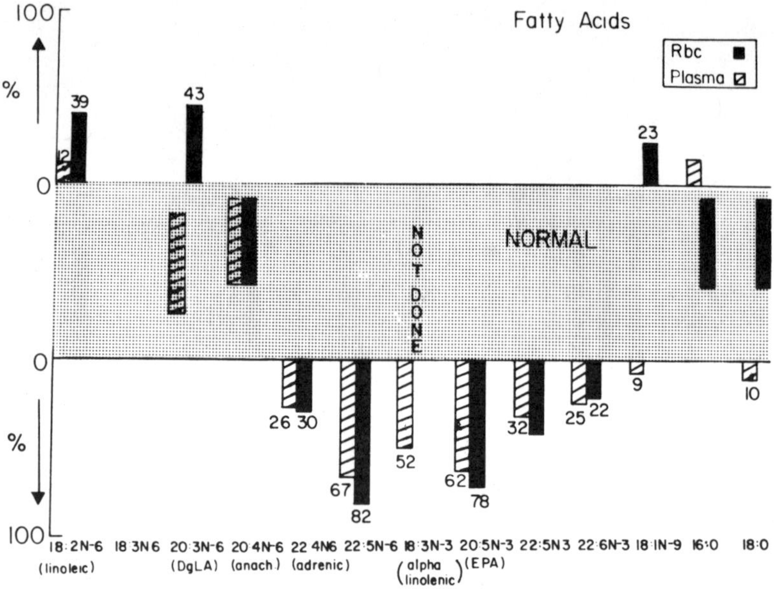

Figure 4:
Percent deviation above or below normal of the average values in 24 untreated patients of individual plasma and Rbc membrane fatty acids.

very complexity of its manifestations is perhaps the greatest single obstacle to acceptance of the concept that Candida albicans may be responsible for chronic illness. The objection voiced most often is that nothing could cause such multi-system illness. This reaction is understandable if human illness is viewed primarily in terms of individual organs and systems, and categorized as "heart trouble," "liver disease," "kidney disease," "stomach trouble," etc.

The most convincing answer to this legitimate reservation would be the demonstration of a mechanism whereby this yeast could interfere simultaneously with the function of several organs. Next would be the finding of abnormalities in blood or urine of patients presenting the typical symptoms of this condition, with the coincidental disappearance of symptoms and laboratory abnormalities with treatment directed at the patient's mold sensitivity.

Evidence of the latter type is suggested in the results of this study. Abnormalities were found in the blood and urine of 24 patients with mold sensitivity, including difficulty resisting yeast overgrowth. When these studies were repeated in seven of the 24 patients following significant clinical improvement, a striking trend to or toward normal was found in abnormalities that were present before treatment.

Evidence of the former type is not yet forthcoming, but the acetaldehyde hypothesis proposes such a biochemical mechanism — one by which to relate the metabolism of Candida albicans to symptoms induced by its overgrowth in the human body. If verifiable, a means will have been found by which this yeast can cause symptoms that are not restricted by the anatomical boundaries that, at least in part, determine the names of most diseases. The disease "pellagra" illustrates this principle. Medical students learn

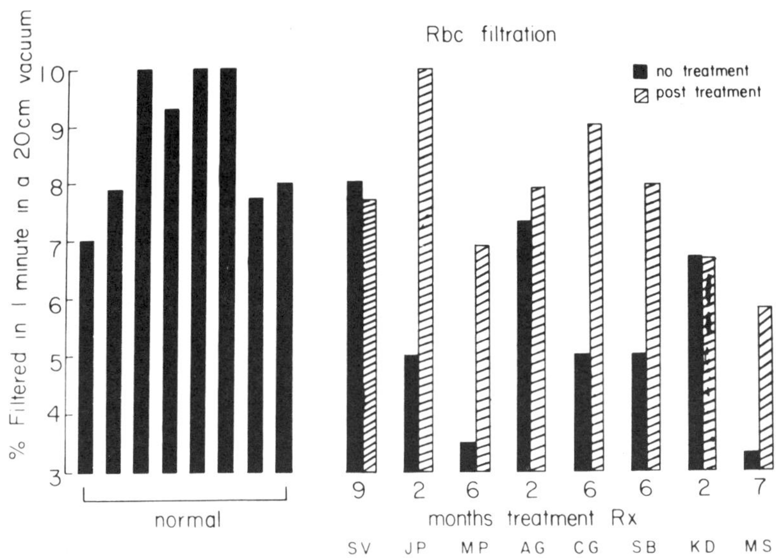

Figure 5:
Red blood cell filtration values of 8 healthy adults as compared with the filtration rate of 8 patients with candidiasis. The solid bars represent filtration values of controls and of patients before treatment. Hatched bars represent values of patients after treatment. The figures under each bar show the number of months of treatment for each patient.

"the three D's" (diarrhea, dermatitis, dementia) of this illness caused by Vitamin B_3 deficiency. The intestine, brain, and skin are manifesting abnormal function because, even though widely separated anatomically, they share metabolic pathways that require adequate B_3.

At the beginning of these studies, only amino acid and fatty acid determinations were available. Rbc filtration was added somewhat later. Specific studies of carbohydrate metabolism were the last to be incorporated into the study and will be reported separately. Indirect but suggestive evidence of interference in carbohydrate pathways will be discussed in connection with the amino acid abnormalities found in these 24 patients.

The finding of abnormalities in all three areas studied increases the likelihood of their significance. It also greatly lessens the chance of these findings being invalid because of errors in the normal control values. While regional differences in such factors as diet and climate could conceivably affect "normal" values, it is quite improbable that this would occur in all three aspects of this investigation, particularly in view of the wide geographic separation of the three laboratories participating in the study.

Among these abnormal results are certain findings worthy of special comment. These will be discussed briefly, with emphasis on changes consistent with those that have been reported among the toxic effects of acetaldehyde.

Fatty Acids

First, in the omega 6 (W-6) series of fatty acids in Rbc membranes, the levels of the shorter chain 18:2W-6 (linoleic acid) and

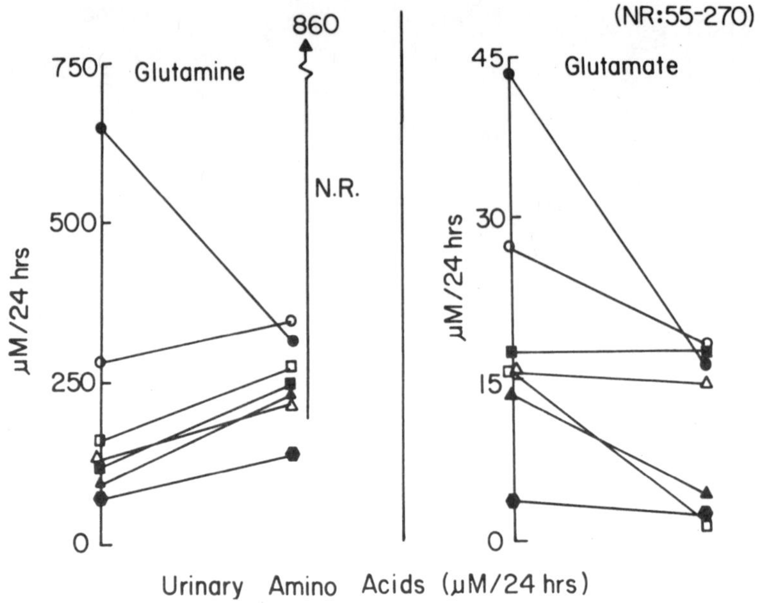

Figure 6:
Changes in urinary excretion of glutamate and glutamine in seven candidiasis patients, after treatment of two to nine months. The symbols on the ends of the lines identify individual patients.

20:3W-6 (DGLA) were elevated, while the longer chain fatty acids 22:4W-6 and 22:5W-6 were below normal. This suggests an impairment of the elongation reaction for which acetyl CoA furnishes the two-carbon units. As we have seen, acetaldehyde inhibits the formation of acetyl CoA.

In the omega 3 series (W-3) the amount of each of the three fatty acids studied was significantly below normal. Rudin believes that most modern diets are deficient in alpha linolenic acid, the precursor of the W-3 series of fatty acids (Rudin, 1983). There is no reason to believe, however, that in this respect the diet in the control patients was different from that of these 24 patients. Even should the values considered "normal" be below optimum because of inadequate dietary alpha linolenic acid, the levels in these patients still were well below that of the controls.

24-hour Amino Acid Excretion

Turning next to an examination of the pattern of amino acid excretion in the urine, we find a number of abnormalities, as shown in Table I. The general picture is one of reduced excretion of many individual amino acids, although in certain instances excretion is above normal.

The excretion of glutamate and glutamine was generally quite low. These two amino acids are widely involved in metabolic pathways, particularly as the principal amine donors in transamination reactions. Glutamine is derived from glutamate, which also is the precursor of GABA (gamma amino butyric acid). GABA is thought to be an inhibitory neurotransmitter. If its formation

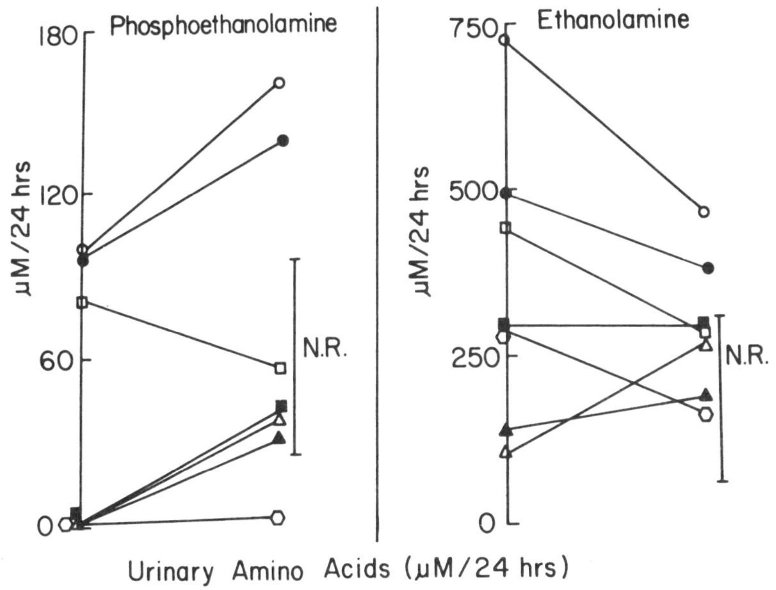

Figure 7:
Changes in urinary excretion of ethanolamine and phosphoethanolamine in seven candidiasis patients, with p values for those that are abnormal.

is impaired because of a decrease in available glutamate, this could be partly responsible for CNS symptoms that often occur in the yeast syndrome.

Analysis of normal brain tissue has shown an abundance of glutamic acid, glutamine, aspartic acid, N acetylaspartic acid, ethanolamine, taurine, cystathionine, glutathione, and asparagine (West, 1975). Glutamic and aspartic acids and their derivatives constitute about 70 percent of non-nitrogenous nitrogen of the brain. Aspartic acid is converted into asparagine, which was extremely low in the urine of these patients. As stated earlier, the finding of increased excretion of ethanolamine in association with reduced excretion of phosphoethanolamine suggests an impairment of this interconversion. The presence of both amines in brain tissue suggests that this conversion normally takes place there also.

Repeat Studies

In the patients thus far restudied, it is important to note that the very low glutamine levels have risen sharply, reaching normal in three and rising from 69 to 134 (normal is 140) in the fourth. Further, an impressive fall in ethanolamine correlated well with a rise in phosphoethanolamine, suggesting removal of the previous block in this interconversion. At this point in treatment asparagine showed no significant change.

Acetaldehyde impairs protein synthesis and secretion. Its binding to amine groups in Schiff base formation could interfere with transamination reactions involved in the synthesis of non-essential amino acids. Also, if by inhibition of acetyl CoA it depressed the citric acid cycle, acetaldehyde could induce a deficiency of the citric acid cycle intermediates that furnish the carbon skeletons of the non-essential amino acids. Thus it is

PLASMA PHOSPHOLIPIDS

FATTY ACID	NORMAL	CANDIDA	
18:2n-6	21.45 ± 2.81	24.96 ± 4.5	*
18:3n-6	0.16 ± 0.12	------	
20:3n-6	3.06 ± 0.60	3.04 ± 0.91	
20:4n-6	11.36 ± 1.67	11.57 ± 2.27	
22:4n-6	0.73 ± 0.26	0.54 ± 0.24	*
22:5n-6	1.12 ± 0.67	0.36 ± 0.21	**
18:3n-3	0.27 ± 0.53	0.13 ± 0.15	*
20:5n-3	1.01 ± 0.36	0.38 ± 0.37	**
22:5n-3	0.93 ± 0.27	0.02 ± 0.28	**
22:6n-3	3.54 ± 0.89	2.67 ± 1.01	**
18:1n-9	13.50 ± 2.20	12.29 ± 1.50	*
16:0	25.81 ± 1.69	29.41 ± 2.19	**
18:0	11.61 ± 1.32	10.43 ± 1.67	*

* = $p < 0.05$
** = $p < 0.01$ or less

Table III:
Average plasma phospholipid values in normal healthy adults and in 24 patients with candidiasis, with p values for those that are abnormal. Expressed as area percent of total phospholipids.

possible, theoretically, to relate acetaldehyde to the amino acid abnormalities found in these patients.

The trend toward normal of the pattern of amino acid excretion was associated with a similar trend in fatty acid balance both in plasma and in Rbc membranes. The very low levels of 22:5W6 fatty acids became normal as their shorter-chain precursors fell from elevated pre-treatment levels, suggesting a correction of the previous impairment of elongation.

Changes in fatty acids of the W-3 series were mixed, some decreasing and others increasing. A 40 percent increase occurred in the average of the value of 22:6W3. Whether this rise will continue must await later determinations.

As stated earlier, acetaldehyde will increase the rigidity of erythrocyte membranes, and has been used for that purpose by physiologists studying membrane composition and function. In patients with chronic candidiasis, diminished flexibility of Rbc membranes resulted in a decrease in filterability of intact red blood cells. This is an important finding, both as a potential diagnostic test, and for its implications in the patho-physiology of this illness.

The return to normal of Rbc filtration was striking in patients whose symptoms simultaneously showed substantial improvement. Improved oxygenation of tissues suggests itself as an important factor in this clinical improvement, particularly of those symptoms related to brain function.

RED BLOOD CELL TOTAL PHOSPHOLIPIDS

FATTY ACID	NORMAL + SD	CANDIDA		
18:2n-6	9.78 ± 1.64	13.63 ± 4.78	Linoleic	**
20:3n-6	1.37 ± 0.37	1.96 ± 0.52	DGLA	**
20:4n-6	15.13 ± 1.98	15.73 ± 3.35	Arachidonic	
22:4n-6	5.54 ± 1.37	3.89 ± 1.02	Adrenic	**
22:5n-6	3.99 ± 1.85	0.73 ± 0.45		**
20:5n-3	0.65 ± 0.24	0.14 ± 0.18	EPA	**
22:5n-3	2.53 ± 0.90	1.45 ± 0.68		**
22:6n-3	4.20 ± 1.03	3.26 ± 0.89		**
18:1n-9	14.83 ± 1.69	18.25 ± 2.46	Oleic	**
16:0	20.68 ± 1.54	21.31 ± 2.18	Palmitic	
18:0	14.71 ± 1.52	16.04 ± 2.86	Stearic	

* = p < 0.05
** = p < 0.01 or less

Table IV:
Average erythrocyte phospholipids in normal healthy adults and in 24 patients with candidiasis, with p values for those that are abnormal. Expressed as area percent of total phospholipids.

Speculation about Membranes and Chronic Candidiasis

Membrane physiology has attracted much attention in recent years. The great importance of membranes in normal physiologic processes is generally accepted. In addition to demarcating its boundaries, membranes compartmentalize the different functions of the cell and its subdivisions, and control the passage of substances involved in its various metabolic processes. Molecules pass in both directions through membranes that also define such anatomical limits as those of the cell nucleus, the mitochondrion, and the cell itself. Passage may be passive or active. Changes in the chemical and physical properties of membranes may alter such transport, resulting in abnormal function of the cell, and ultimately of its parent organ.

Numerous membrane pumps and shunts function in metabolic pathways. Several examples illustrate their importance in normal cellular function. (1) NADH formed in the cytoplasm during glycolysis cannot cross the mitochondrial membrane for reconversion to NAD, without which glycolysis cannot proceed. Cytoplasmic NAD is regenerated by the transfer of hydrogen from NADH to glycerol 3-phosphate or to malate, both of which are able to cross the mitochondrial membrane. Thus, in addition to assuring a continuous supply of NAD in the cytoplasm, these "shuttles" accomplish the necessary transfer of hydrogen into the mitochondria, where, by oxidative phosphorylation and the electron transport chain, it is ultimately accepted by molecular oxygen as ATP is formed. (2) The reciprocal transport of ADP and ATP across the inner mitochondrial membrane requires the specific carrier, "ATP-ADP translocase." (3) In fatty acid oxidation, carnitine carries acyl groups across the inner mitochondrial membrane to the mitochondrial matrix, in which oxidation takes place. (4) Gluconeogenesis takes place in the cytoplasm, where are located the glycolytic enzymes that catalyze the formation of glycogen from pyruvate, and from amino acids that have first been converted to oxaloacetate. However, the formation of oxaloacete from amino acids occurs in the mitochondria, and oxaloacete is unable to cross the mitochondrial membrane into the cytoplasm; to do so it must be converted to malate, which, once in the cytoplasm, is reconverted to oxalacetate. Thus gluconeogenesis is dependent on the proper passage of malate through the mitochondrial membrane. (5) Glycolysis takes place in the cytoplasm, but the further oxidation of carbohydrate is by the citric acid cycle and oxidative phosphorylation, both of which occur in the mitochondrion. Therefore pyruvate must be transported from the cytoplasm into the mitochondria by the "pyruvate carrier," (6) Steroid hormones, after passing through cell walls from serum, bind to appropriate receptor proteins in the cytoplasm and are carried into the nucleus, where they exert their normal modulating effect on cell function. (7) Electrical conductance and normal function in nerve and muscle tissue depend upon the movement across membranes of such ions as sodium, potassium, and calcium. Such transmembrane proteins as Na^{+}-K^{+} ATPase and Ca^{++} ATPase, as they are alternately phosphorylated and dephosphorylated, undergo configurational changes that are vital to their function. The importance of these two pumps needs no emphasis. Membrane abnormalities sufficient to impair their efficient operation would have far-reaching effects on normal physiologic processes. For example, the movement into the cell of such metabolic fuels as glucose and amino acids is often tied to the movement of Na^{+}, which is driven by the N^{+}-K^{+} pump. (8) Other transport systems of the mitochondrial membrane include the dicarboxylate and tricarboxylate carriers for transporting citric acid cycle intermediates, the glutamate carrier, and a transport system for calcium ions.

These few examples illustrate the importance of properly regulated passage of metabolic intermediates, minerals, and electrolytes into and out of the cell and its various compartments. It is difficult to conceive of pathways that would remain unaffected by major membrane abnormalities.

In these candidiasis patients abnormalities of fatty acid balance in serum and Rbc membranes occurred consistently, in association with impaired filterability of these cells. Although at this time we do not know whether these cell-wall abnormalities extend to cells other than erythrocytes, it would seem more probable than not, in view of the fact that the same imbalance of fatty acids was found in serum as in red cell membranes. This is a matter of great importance.

Acetaldehyde may affect Rbc membranes directly, or it may do so by metabolic interference that leads to imbalances of fatty acids and other membrane constituents. Either effect of this toxin could be exerted on membranes elsewhere in the body, affecting some perhaps more than others. It is interesting, as part of the acetaldehyde hypothesis, to speculate about the possible relationship of such membrane changes to some of the clinical manifestations of chronic candidiasis in patients with mold sensitivity and the associated susceptibility of yeast infections.

Membranes and Gastro-Intestinal Function

The absorption of nutrients would hardly proceed normally if the walls of the cells of the intestinal mucosa were abnormal with respect to permeability and transport. Indeed, even the digestion that must precede the absorption of many nutrients might well be affected if enzyme formation and release were impaired as a result of changes in the cells responsible for these functions.

Acetaldehyde has been shown to have a different effect on intestinal microvillus membrane vesicles than on Rbc membranes (Tillotson et al., 1981). These studies indicated an increase in the fluidity of these membranes, with an associated dissipation of the Na+ gradient, and an inhibition of carrier function. These studies indicated that the permeability of these membranes increased upon exposure to acetaldehyde. Thus, at least in this one instance, acetaldehyde affected membranes by increasing rather than decreasing their fluidity, but in so doing definitely altered vital membrane functions.

Table V

24-HOUR URINE AMINO ACID DETERMINATIONS BEFORE AND AFTER TREATMENT

AMINO ACIDS	NORMAL VALUES	J.W. B	J.W. A	S.B. B	S.B. A	C.G. B	C.G. A	M.P. B	M.P. A	J.P. B	J.P. A	A.G. B	A.G. A	S.V. B	S.V. A
TAURINE	63-2300	726	850	171	42	200	99	281	235	391	407	282	637	656	934
PHOSPHOETHANOLAMINE	26-101	100	163	TR	37	TR	31	TR	41	80	56	TR	TR	97	138
ASPARTIC	23-218	130	102	88	79	132	91	132	135	65	90	207	53	188	151
THREONINE	85-440	71	158	34	59	60	56	237	105	30	71	65	51	104	129
SERINE	160-700	192	380	164	215	117	105	885	347	154	260	246	219	330	455
ASPARAGINE	270-700	60	65	3	49	28	37	105	53	64	42	50	28	45	38
GLUTAMIC ACID	55-270	16	3	7	4	12	8	27	21	16	14	20	20	42	17
A-AMINOADIPIC ACID	31-81	8	56	18	27	14	18	10	22	TR	21	TR	12	TR	30
GLYCINE	160-4200	872	1492	262	395	1041	547	8613	3538	839	1710	1200	1164	2291	2467
GLUTAMINE	140-860	122	246	69	135	130	216	650	317	92	229	161	269	282	341
ALANINE	60-800	255	328	37	86	177	99	802	335	57	160	96	134	347	287
A-AMINO N-BUTYRIC	16-77	19	21	13	17	16	32	69	62	8	35	21	29	38	48
VALINE	14-51	22	27	9	16	18	16	31	27	TR	15	18	16	16	34
CYSTINE	20-130	83	55	57	52	66	52	255	85	37	49	115	71	138	120
METHIONINE	20-95	16	37	12	23	12	18	38	40	13	28	31	46	29	44
CYSTATHIONINE	16-63	16	22	TR	TR	TR	TR	TR	11	7	TR	TR	18	12	TR
ISOLEUCINE	18-210	15	34	TR	11	14	24	TR	9	4	7	8	31	10	9
LEUCINE	21-200	26	36	10	18	20	20	26	27	7	14	19	36	26	27
TYROSINE	40-270	67	59	12	20	58	41	128	55	17	34	45	42	65	58
PHENYLALANINE	24-190	67	27	17	27	28	20	228	*	105	26	32	27	218	*
ETHANOLAMINE	59-307	139	188	285	169	295	293	438	280	105	264	724	463	492	380
LYSINE	48-640	119	113	36	27	50	50	589	218	19	42	153	149	121	177
L-METHYLHISTIDINE	130-930	54	513	279	47	33	43	425	513	16	26	80	54	54	62
HISTIDINE	130-2100	688	675	116	214	227	164	1164	620	97	187	266	324	417	513
3-METHYLHISTIDINE	56-249	226	292	173	174	174	180	333	209	104	181	267	226	281	341

*unable to calculate due to interfering substance

Table V: Urinary amino acid levels in 7 patients before and after treatment of chronic candidasis. Expressed in MCM/24 hours.

Table VI

Plasma Fatty Acids

	Average values of five patients		Normal range
18:1N9	before after	11.82 16.27	11.3 - 15.7
18:2N6	before after	25.83 22.47	18.6 - 24.3
20:3N6	before after	3.06 3.23	2.5 - 3.7
20:4N6	before after	10.77 12.08	9.7 - 13.0
22:4N6	before after	0.46 0.63	0.47 - 0.99
22:5N6	before after	0.36 0.51	0.45 - 1.8
20:5N3	before after	0.47 0.36	0.65 - 1.4
22:5N3	before after	0.72 0.63	0.66 - 1.2
22:6N3	before after	2.52 2.68	2.6 - 4.4

Table VI:
Average of individual values in five patients before and after treatment for each of nine fatty acids. Expressed as area percent of total phospholipids.

Table VII

Red Blood Cell Membrane Fatty Acids

	Average patient values		Normal range
18:1N9	before after	17.65 16.83	13.14 - 16.52
18:2N6	before after	16.16 10.93	8.14 - 11.42
20:3N6	before after	2.05 1.83	1.0 - 1.74
20:4N6	before after	16.4 16.9	13.15 - 17.11
22:4N6	before after	4.11 4.19	4.17 - 6.91
22:5N6	before after	0.96 1.13	2.14 - 5.84
20:5N3	before after	0.20 0.28	0.41 - 0.89
22:5N3	before after	1.78 1.69	1.63 - 3.43
22:6N3	before after	3.11 3.81	3.17 - 5.23

Table VII:
Average of nine individual fatty acids in the Rbc membranes of five patients before and after treatment. Expressed as area percent of total phospholipids.

Membranes and Lymphocyte Function

Membranes are uniquely important in the function of lymphocytes. The many complex events involved in their function follow the initial recognition of markers on the surface of target cells by appropriate sites on the membranes of the lymphocyte itself. This is important both in triggering the normal response to "foreign" antigens, and in preventing the abnormal attacks of "self" antigens that lead to "auto-immune" disease. Abnormalities of the membranes of lymphocytes should have an effect on both functions.

An impaired response to foreign antigens should weaken the attack on Candida albicans itself, such a condition of "immunologic tolerance" being borne out by the chronic, resistant nature of infections with this yeast. It could also weaken our immunologic defense against other microorganisms, and perhaps even against malignant cells. On the other hand, failure to properly recognize "self" antigens could result in ineffective suppression, with resulting immunologic responses to normal cells, immune-complex deposition, and autoimmune disease.

There is another way that membrane changes could result in autoimmune disease. Should such changes in cells other than lymphocytes lead to exposure of antigenic determinants that are normally hidden (e.g., the hydrophobic portion of a membrane protein), lymphocytes might then falsely recognize as "foreign" these "new" markers. Thus autoimmune attacks could result (1) when lymphocyte function is normal, but hidden antigens become exposed or, (2) when lymphocyte function is abnormal and suppressor function fails, allowing attacks on antigens that are normally exposed.

Certain characteristics of autoimmune reactions are more easily explained by the second hypothesis, i.e., that antigenic determinants normally hidden are exposed as a result of membrane damage. First, in autoimmune illness the attacks are directed at different organs, so that different "diseases" occur among such patients. Second, often more than one autoimmune "disease" is present simultaneously in the same patient, even though one usually predominates. This variability in the intensity of autoimmune attacks is readily explained by the hypothesis that membranes of different organs vary in their degree of abnormality, and hence of exposed "hidden" determinants. Suppressor cell weakness alone, in the absence of any "strange" antigens, should lead to attacks more nearly equal in intensity in the various organs.

As stated earlier, it would be likely that both mechanisms would be involved, since membrane abnormality, if widespread, would involve suppressor lymphocytes, as well as the cells of the organs under attack.

Membranes and Erythrocyte Function

Turning now to erythrocytes, we can anticipate that the increased rigidity of their membranes would render these cells less able to accomplish the changes in shape and fluidity necessary for passage through capillaries one-third their own diameter. If this should affect oxygenation of an organ, it would impair its function. The brain, for example, is highly susceptible to even slight reductions in oxygen tension, this being manifested particularly as an impairment of short-term memory, a symptom characteristically seen in these patients (Davis and Berger, 1979).

The "anion channel" of the Rbc membrane is another example of the importance of membrane integrity in regulating the movement of ions and molecules across membranes. The anion channel is a glycoprotein that traverses the Rbc membrane, all molecules pointing in the same direction. It accounts for about 20-30 percent of Rbc membrane protein. This channel allows the passage of Cl^- and HCO_3^- through the Rbc membrane as erythrocytes transport CO_2. A decrease in the normal fluidity of the Rbc membrane, as found in these patients, could affect the conformational changes necessary for the proper function of such a protein pump.

Special Problems in Patients with Chronic Candidiasis

In patients with mold sensitivity and yeast susceptibility, several problems occur at a frequency greater than expected in the general population.

Mitral Valve Prolapse

The first of these is mitral valve prolapse with dysautonomia. The medical history usually reveals that the symptoms on which these diagnoses were based had their beginning after typical symptoms of mold sensitivity had been present for several years. If we assume that these conditions are being diagnosed with reasonable accuracy, there has been a sharp increase in their incidence, and it has paralleled the similar increase that has occurred in chronic yeast infections since the advent of broad-spectrum antibiotics, birth-control pills, and steroid hormones.

Carpal Tunnel Syndrome

Another condition that has been seen with some frequency in this syndrome is carpal tunnel syndrome. The effects of acetaldehyde, especially that on collagen metabolism, could be related to this and to the mitral valve prolapse problem.

Formaldehyde Sensitivity

Many of these patients exhibit extreme intolerance to formaldehyde. Since it also binds to sulfhydryl and amine groups, and in general exhibits toxicity similar to that of acetaldehyde, the effects of these two aldehydes should be additive. A patient whose tissues already contained a significant amount of acetaldehyde might well exhibit symptoms from an amount of formaldehyde that otherwise would be easily tolerated. In addition, aldehyde dehydrogenase oxidizes both toxins. The requirement for the continuous removal of acetaldehyde should to some degree diminish the capacity of the liver to cope with formaldehyde. Thus the hypothesis of acetaldehyde toxicity could account for what has been one of the most puzzling aspects of this illness.

Occasionally patients date the onset of this illness to heavy formaldehyde exposure. Such an event could be superimposed on mild acetaldehyde toxicity (i.e., mild candidiasis), or indeed, might theoretically initiate the problem, which would then be perpetuated by acetaldehyde despite the elimination of further exposure to formaldehyde. In fact, once the membrane (and metabolic) abnormalities have been initiated by either aldehyde, according to this hypothesis the resulting impairment of lymphocyte function would allow further growth of Candida albicans. As this occurred, acetaldehyde would be produced in increasing quantities, to perpetuate and advance the illness.

Careful histories frequently relate the onset of yeast susceptibility to such yeast-stimulating factors as antibiotics and contraceptive hormones, indicating that in these cases acetaldehyde initiated the aldehyde toxicity. In theory, however, heavy and prolonged formaldehyde exposure could start the process. The practical fact is that formaldehyde exposure in the usual amount tolerated by healthy individuals would almost always be present as an additional factor in patients, even as the process was being initiated by acetaldehyde.

End-Organ Response to Hormones

Another important category of symptoms in these patients includes manifestations suggestive of impaired end-organ responsiveness to hormones, especially the steroid hormones. For example, severe menstrual bleeding and poor vaginal cornification may occur despite normal blood levels of ovarian hormones.

The functional state of membranes could influence the cell's response to hormones. In order to exert their proper physiologic effect, steroid hormones must pass through the cell wall, and then through the nuclear membrane. Insulin and similar membrane-active hormones bind to receptors on cell walls. Should membrane changes affect the entry of steroid hormones into the cytoplasm or nucleus, or alter the insulin receptor so as to affect its binding, these hormones could be hindered in exerting their normal effect on the cell. It is just such an impairment of the cellular response to hormones that is suggested by many of the symptoms in this syndrome.

Autonomic Imbalance

Other frequently occurring symptoms are those characteristic of imbalance of the autonomic nervous system. Acetylcholine is the neurotransmitter at both sympathetic and parasympathetic synapses of the autonomic nervous system, and also mediates the action of post-ganglion parasympathetic neurons. Acetaldehyde is a potent synaptic blocking agent and could be responsible for the autonomic imbalance in these patients, perhaps in part by binding to the sulfhydryl group of CoA, thus affecting the availablility of the acetyl group required for the synthesis of acetylcholine.

Central Nervous System Symptoms

Defective short-term memory, also common in patients with this condition, could be another effect of impaired acetylcholine function, brought on either by such poor transacetylation, or by membrane abnormality that affected its release from synaptic vesicles.

Impairment of the ability to concentrate usually accompanies the memory deficit, most often in association with depression and anxiety. The many neurotransmitters that are amines may, by Schiff base formation with acetaldehyde, form "false neurotransmitters." These compounds should have an adverse effect on neuronal function that utilizes these amines as neurotransmitters.

Thus, among the mechanisms by which acetaldehyde theoretically could cause the common symptoms of depression, anxiety, and difficulty with memory and concentration, we have the following:

1. Metabolic disturbances in neurons (fatty acid, protein, carbohydrate)
2. Membrane abnormalities
3. Impairment of acetylcholine synthesis or release
4. Defective neurotransmitter function
    a.) defective synthesis, release, or binding
    b.) false neurotransmitter formation
5. Diminished oxygen delivery due to loss of flexibility of erythrocyte membranes

Allergic Symptoms

Allergic reactions to products of Candida albicans occur frequently. Allergic rhinitis and asthma are not uncommon. Chronic "idiopathic" urticaria is frequently due to the antigens of this yeast.

Whether, or how, the toxic effects of acetaldehyde play a part in the allergic response is not clear. Its effect on membranes could alter the reactivity of cells of the mucous membranes and skin, but this seems less likely than an acetaldehyde-induced change in leukocytes.

At this time too little is known of the changes that occur in leukocytes when they begin to mediate the symptoms of allergy. Theoretically there might have occurred a decrease in a normal function that suppresses this type reaction. Or it could be an entirely new reaction — one that does not occur normally, for which therefore no suppressor mechanisms exist, or are needed. If it affected their metabolism or membranes (or both), theoretically acetaldehyde could alter leukocytes in such a way that they begin to function in this abnormal way.

Two observations are of interest in this regard. Certain patients previously free of allergies have experienced their initial allergic reactions to pollen and other inhalants while receiving long-term antibiotic therapy for acne. The timing of the initial reaction (to pollen, for example) often coincides with the onset of diarrhea, vaginitis, and other manifestations of the yeast problem. Then, in rapid succession, other inhalants and foods begin to trigger the allergic response.

The second observation dates from approximately three years ago. For many years prior to that time there had been no way to test the idea that the effect of Candida albicans on the cells of the immune system might include those changes in lymphocytes (whatever they are) that account for the onset of allergic responses. Withholding standard pollen extract therapy, for example, could not be justified in patients whose history and skin tests clearly indicated Spring and Fall pollen hay fever.

When chronic yeast infections are treated in patients who also have major autoimmune illness, vaccines are not used, since such stimuli to the immune system theoretically might also stimulate its autoimmune component. Thus, even in the presence of severe Spring or Fall pollen hay fever, the usual allergy injections are not used; symptomatic treatment (e.g. antihistamines) is recommended.

Some patients began reporting complete disappearance of these typical pollen symptoms. In some cases, total relief was experienced from both Spring and Fall pollen hay fever symptoms, even though symptoms in both seasons had been severe for many consecutive years. This simultaneous remission (i.e., in the same year) of tree and/or grass hay fever in the Spring, and ragweed hay fever in the Fall, virtually insures that the responsible change was in the patient rather than in the environment. This occurrence suggests a relationship between Candida albicans and the functional abnormality of the immune system that is associated with this type of allergy response.

Thus both observations — that allergies to pollen, other inhalants, and foods may appear in quick succession soon after the onset of chronic yeast infections, and on occasion may disappear abruptly with no therapy other than yeast suppression — suggest a relationship between Candida albicans and the unknown changes in the immune system that allow (or cause) allergic reactions to occur. How often this might be true remains to be determined.

It has also proved true that in some cases of intractable asthma, the addition of yeast suppression has led to sudden improvement beyond that achieved by extract therapy. This may mean only that certain yeast substances were among the antigens to which the patient was allergic. However, considered in conjunction with the two observations just discussed, it suggests that the benefit may possibly have resulted from an effect of nystatin on some factor more basic to the allergic mechanism.

Summary

The results of metabolic studies in 24 patients with chronic candidiasis have been presented. An attempt has been made to consider the principal symptoms of this condition, and these metabolic findings, in relation to various toxic effects of acetaldehyde. Though speculative, these thoughts as to how this toxin could cause the clinical and laboratory characteristics of this illness are a vital part of this hypothesis. The extensive literature on the subject of acetaldehyde provides a number of mechanisms by which its toxicity could lead to this illness, and to the abnormal laboratory results reported in this paper.

The appeal of the acetaldehyde hypothesis is that it defines the symptoms of chronic yeast infection in terms of a toxin that is readily produced in vitro by common strains of Candida albicans. It provides the needed chemical link between normal yeast fermentation and metabolic abnormalities in patients with yeast susceptibility.

Indirect evidence indicates that, in vivo, Candida albicans ferments sugars to acetaldehyde. Final proof of this hypothesis will require direct evidence to that effect.

References

AMMON, H.P.T. et al.: Effect of Alcohol and Acetaldehyde on Coenzyme A. In: The Biological Aspects of Alcohol. Roach, Mary K. (ed), University of Texas Press, 185-211, 1971.

AMMON, H.P.T. et al.: Inactivation of Coenzyme A by Ethanol: Acetaldehyde as Mediator of the Inactivation of Coenzyme A Following the Administration of Ethanol In Vivo. Biochem. Pharmacol. 18, 29-33, 1969.

BARKER, S.B.: Acetaldehyde in Mammalian Red Blood Cells. J. Biol. Chem. 137, 783-784, 1941.

COHEN, G. and COLLINS. M.A.: Alkaloids from Catecholamines in Adrenal Tissue: Possible Role in Alcoholism. Science 167, 1749-1751, 1970.

DAVIS, K.L. and BERGER, P.A. (eds): Brain Acetylcholine and Neuropsychiatric Disease. Plenum Press, 1979.

DAVIS, W.E. and WALSH, M.J.: Alcohol, Amines, and Alkaloids: A Possible Biochemical Basis for Alcohol Addiction. Science 167, 1005-1007, 1970.

GAINES, K.C. et al.: Reaction of Acetaldehyde with Human Erythrocyte Membrane Proteins. FEBS Letters 75, 115-121, 1977.

IWATA, K.: Proceedings of Second International Specialized Symposium on Yeasts, Tokyo, 1972.

LIEBER, C.S.: Metabolism and Metabolic Effects of Alcohol. Seminars in Hematology 17, 85-99, 1980.

LUMENG, L. and TING-KAI LI: Vitamin B_6 in Chronic Alcohol Abuse: Pyridoxal Phosphate Levels in Plasma and the Effects of Acetaldehyde on Pyridoxal Phosphate Synthesis and Degradation in Human Erythrocytes. J. of Clin. Invest. 53, 693-704, 1974.

PALMER, A.A. and BETTS, W.H.: The Axial Drift of Fresh and Acetaldehyde-Hardened Erythrocytes in 25 mm Capillary Slits of Various Lengths. Biorheology 12, 283-292, 1975.

RUDIN, D.O.: The Three Pellagras. Journal of Orthomolecular Psychiatry 12, 91-110, 1983.

SANDLER, M. et al.: Tetrahydroisoquinoline Alkaloids: In Vivo Metabolites of L-DOPA in Man. Nature 241, 439-443, 1973.

TILLOTSON, C.G. et al.: Inhibition of Na^+-Stimulated Glucose Transport Function and Perturbation of Intestinal Microvillus Membrane Vesicles by Ethanol and Acetaldehyde. Arch. Biochem. and Biophysics 207, 360-370, 1981.

TRUSS, C.O.: Clinical Observations on Candida Albicans. Paper presented at the Eighth Scientific Symposium, Academy of Orthomolecular Psychiatry, Toronto, 1977.

TRUSS, C.O.: Restoration of Immunologic Competence to Candida Albicans. Journal of Orthomolecular Psychiatry 9, 287-301, 1980.

TRUSS, C.O.: Tissue Injury Induced by Candida Albicans: Mental and Neurologic Manifestations. Journal of Orthomolecular Psychiatry 7, 17-37, 1978.

TRUSS, C.O.: The Missing Diagnosis. P.O. Box 26508, Birmingham, AL 35226, 1983.

TRUSS, C.O.: The Role of Candida Albicans in Human Illness. Journal of Orthomolecular Psychiatry 10, 228-238, 1981.

VAN NIEL, C.B. and ANDERSON, E.H.: On the Occurrence of Fermentative Assimilation. J. Cell and Comp. Physiol. 17, 49-56, 1941.

VAN NIEL, C.B. and COHEN, A.L.: On the Metabolism of Candida Albicans. J. Cell. Comp. Physiol. 20, 95-112, 1942.

VASSAR, P.S. et al.: Physicochemical Effects of Aldehydes on the Human Erythrocyte. J. Cell Bio. 53, 809-818, 1972.

VEITCH, R. et al.: Vitamin B_6 Metabolism in Chronic Alcohol Abuse: Effect of Ethanol Oxidation on Hepatic Pyridoxal 5'-Phosphate Metabolism. J. Clin. Invest. 55, 1026-1032, 1975.

WEST, E.: Textbook of Biochemistry. 4th ed., Macmillan Co. p. 1317-1319, 1975.

Journal of Advancement in Medicine
Volume 5, Number 3, Fall 1992

Generalized Symptoms in Women with Chronic Yeast Vaginitis: Treatment with Nystatin, Diet and Immunotherapy Versus Nystatin Alone

C. Orian Truss, MD, Carroll V. Truss, PhD, and Robert B. Cutler, PhD

ABSTRACT: It has been proposed that superficial Candida albicans infections of the vagina and gastrointestinal tract may cause a variety of generalized symptoms. Immediately following a 32-week study of partial treatment with 4 nystatin/placebo regimens, 25 pre-menopausal women with chronic yeast vaginitis received 26 weeks of full treatment (nystatin, diet, immunotherapy). Full treatment was compared to nystatin/placebo for 3 vaginal and 25 non-vaginal (general) symptoms. Twenty-seven of 28 decreased significantly (10 at $P<.001$, 15 at $P<.02$, 2 at $P<.05$); diarrhea, near zero at week 32, decreased 50% (ns). Improvement was highly significant for vaginal, non-vaginal, and psychological, each at $P<.001$; digit span, $P<.05$. Proportion of patients improving was significant, each at $P<.001$, for vaginal (20 of 25), non-vaginal (25 of 25), and psychological (24 of 25, one patient already normal at week 32 baseline remaining so). For digit-span (DS), 13 of 18 initially scoring below 13 (norm is 10) improved; none of the 5 initially above 12 improved. Degree of improvement was significantly correlated with week 32 scores for all 4 categories. Limited treatment for the first 32 weeks with 4 nystatin/placebo regimens reduced 24 of 25 general symptoms (unlikely by chance, $P<.0000008$ by exact probability); four reached significance. Full treatment, weeks 32-58, lead to highly significant and clinically relevant *further* improvement, again in 24 of 25 general symptoms. Toxic, immunologic, enzymatic and allergic mechanisms are suggested. A therapeutic trial of nystatin and diet will establish the diagnosis in 6 weeks or less.

C. Orian Truss, M.D., is Medical Director, Critical Illness Research Foundation, Birmingham, Alabama; Carroll V. Truss, Ph.D., is Professor Emeritus, University of Miami (FL), and Robert B. Cutler, Ph.D., is affiliated with the University of Miami (Florida).

Address reprint requests to C. Orian Truss, M.D., Critical Illness Research Foundation, 2614 Highland Avenue, Birmingham, Alabama 35205-1799.

Introduction

> "The principal prerequisite for diagnosis of a disease is that a physician should acknowledge the possibility of its existence" (Odds F.C.) (1).

Chronic candidiasis may be as minimal as a yeast infection under a single nail. Such superficial yeast infections (muco-cutaneous candidiasis) may, however, involve extensive areas of skin as well as the mucous membranes of the vagina and gastrointestinal (GI) tract. These represent the minimum and maximum of chronic candidiasis when yeast infections are limited to these external and internal surfaces of the human body.

Strong opposition has been expressed to the proposal that, at some point along this spectrum from asymptomatic nail infection to widespread involvement of the superficial tissues, generalized symptoms may begin to appear in addition to the local symptoms at the infected sites (2). Representative of this expressed opposition are a number of papers (3-10), none of which have reported failure to confirm the effect of anti-yeast treatment on generalized symptoms, and which therefore represent only opinion. In 1989 the *FDA Consumer* (11), possibly influenced largely by these opinion papers, included "chronic candidiasis" among its list of leading "health frauds."

At the same time, a very large number of patients, when treated for yeast infection in the recommended way (12), are telling their physicians (13-16) that this treatment has proved to be the answer to severe, long-standing health problems in which a variety of general symptoms are described in association with chronic superficial yeast infections. Almost always ultimately dismissed as psychoneuroses, these chronic illnesses typically have been responsible for the expenditure of very large sums of money in repeated but futile efforts to establish an organic basis for the numerous symptoms.

Such passionate opposition to an innocuous and relatively inexpensive treatment needs to be examined, and the controversy settled. The current repetitious application of expensive diagnostic procedures (particularly intestinal x-rays and endoscopies, MRI, and various scans), the numerous consultations and prescription drugs employed to investigate and treat the individual symptoms, and in particular the frequent hospitalizations—make a significant contribution to the cost of medical care.

Patients report long-lasting relief of a variety of general symptoms when nystatin and diet are used to suppress C. albicans (2, 12-18). Is this a placebo effect (unique its permanency) in psychoneurotics, or are the symptoms disappearing because nystatin destroys much of the excess intestinal and vaginal yeast, while diet inhibits the remainder?

As noted, chronic candidiasis that is limited to skin and mucous membranes may be only an asymptomatic infection of a single nail, or be so widespread as to involve much of the skin and mucous membranes of the vagina and GI tract. At issue is whether there is a point along this spectrum beyond which the quantity of yeast and the extent of its penetration into the skin and mucous membranes, and therefore the quantity of yeast products released into the human bloodstream, is such that general ("remote" or "non-local") symptoms begin to appear. These symptoms may include fatigue, inappropriate depression, insomnia or hypersomnia, panic attacks, short-term memory loss and decreased ability to concentrate, decreased libido, menstrual abnormalities, premenstrual tension (PMS), acne, intolerance to environmental chemicals.

In the answer to two questions lies the resolution of this controversy: (1) Is C. albicans, when present in the skin and mucous membranes in sufficient quantity, capable of causing patients to feel bad generally, or is it unique among infectious agents in that there is no limit to the amount that may be present in the mucous membranes without its causing the appearance of such general (non-local) symptoms? Or (2), are these symptoms causing large sums to be spent, often over a span of many years, on non-productive searches for their cause in a very large number of psychoneurotics?

Products produced by C. albicans include antigens as well as non-antigenic toxins. By crossed immunoelectrophoresis, 79 antibodies in human sera were found to react with antigens of C. albicans (19), confirming the release of at least this number of antigens. Toxins produced by C. albicans have been reviewed (5,20-21). These include those with endotoxic and hydrolytic activity (22), acetaldehyde (13,18, 23), arabinotol (24), and canditoxin (20). Thus the potential exists for the production of general symptoms by a variety of mechanisms, both toxic and immunologic (e.g., immune-complex deposition, allergic).

The initial report in 1978 (2) that general symptoms may accompany the usual local symptoms of superficial yeast infections was based on recognition of the simultaneous disappearance of such "non-local" symptoms when the skin and mucosal "local" symptoms were brought under control, and by their simultaneous reappearance with relapse of superficial yeast infections. The measures used to clear the infections, and therefore the measures that led to recognition of the general symptoms that may result from superficial yeast infections, included the antifungal drug nystatin administered orally and vaginally, a low yeast–low carbohydrate diet, immunotherapy when appropriate, and the simultaneous avoidance to the extent possible of factors known to foster the growth of C. albicans in the human body, principally antibiotics, contraceptive hormones, and steroids or other immunosuppressant therapy.

In an effort to evaluate objectively that which was based on clinical observation, The Critical Illness Research Foundation (CIRF)† in 1987 funded a "double blind" study comparing nystatin to placebo in 40 women (51 started) with chronic yeast vaginitis but who also described numerous chronic generalized symptoms. This study was carried out in the Department of Medicine at the Medical College of Alabama (UAB). The results were reported in 1990 (25) (UAB study) and later discussed in our "Letter to the Editor" (26).

Although recommended treatment (12) includes a low yeast–low carbohydrate diet, immunotherapy with C. albicans extract, oral and vaginal nystatin, and avoidance of factors known to foster yeast infections, nystatin was the only component that could be properly blinded. Diet cannot be blinded on a long-term basis, and immunotherapy requires such individualization that blinding it over an extended period is extremely difficult. Thus, the UAB study was a placebo-controlled investigation of nystatin, only one of the three treatment components. Factors that aggravate yeast infections were avoided as much as possible.

Most such blinded studies of a drug are designed to evaluate the effectiveness of the drug as treatment for a particular indication. However, in this instance it was the Foundation's proposal to UAB that we take advantage of the accepted efficacy of nystatin in treating mucosal yeast infections of the vagina and GI tract, to test the validity of the concept that yeast may induce general symptoms in addition to the familiar local symptoms at these sites of mucosal infections. If it could be demonstrated that symptoms of a general nature—symptoms such as fatigue, depression, memory loss, PMS—reappeared and disappeared coincident with symptoms in the vagina (itching, discharge) and in the GI tract (diarrhea, constipation, bloating, nausea, indigestion), as the yeast infection in these two organs

†CIRF -- 2614 Highland Avenue, Birmingham, AL 35205.

waxed and waned when nystatin and placebo were alternated, the validity of this syndrome would have been confirmed.

Definitions

Superficial candidiasis: Yeast infections limited to skin and mucous membranes.

Superficial candidiasis syndrome: superficial yeast infections accompanied by generalized symptoms.

Deep candidiasis: yeast infections of one or more internal organs.

Unless otherwise stated, yeast infection and candidiasis refers to infection with C. albicans.

Materials and Methods

Prior to conclusion of the UAB study in early 1988, the decision was made by the CIRF to compare symptom scores at the end of this study with those after an additional 6 months of uninterrupted FT, to include also diet and immunotherapy. All 40 subjects completing the UAB study were offered the opportunity to begin such full treatment on the same day that each completed that study. At the end of 6 months FT, symptoms were to be re-evaluated by the same two questionnaires and DS test employed in the UAB study.

Of the 40 women completing the UAB study, 39 came for FT. Of these, 27 agreed to meet the stated criteria of (1) six months of uninterrupted FT, beginning on the day that each had completed the UAB study, and (2) self assessment at the end of FT, consisting of completion of the two questionnaires and DS test used and described in the UAB study (25).

The patients that were entered into the UAB study were originally selected and referred by one of us (C.O.T.), using the following criteria: (1) women between the ages of 21 and 40 years; (2) vaginitis that was constant or recurring several times a year, repeatedly diagnosed by each woman's personal physician as yeast-induced, and that had responded consistently to vaginal anti-yeast drugs but with repeated relapses; (3) gastrointestinal symptoms (Table 1); (4) CNS symptoms, including fatigue, depression, poor short-term memory and concentration; (5) menstrual abnormalities including premenstrual tension; (6) respiratory allergies. Each patient had to have had chronic symptoms in each of these categories (Table 1) when selected, although all symptoms were not necessarily present at week 0 of the UAB study. Patients using contraceptive hormones, antibiotics, or immunosuppressant therapy were excluded.

As already indicated, of 40 women completing the UAB study, 39 came for FT, but only 27 met the stated requirements for completing it. Two of these were ultimately excluded for failure to fill in the questionnaires appro-

TABLE 1

Vaginal and Non-Vaginal Symptom Severity Scores, Psychological Measures, and Digit Span for the 25 Full Treatment Patients on Partial (Weeks 0-32) and on Full Treatment (Weeks 32-58)

Week*	0		32		58		Diff.	Confidence	
SYMPTOM	Mean	SD	Mean	SD	Mean	SD	58-32	Interval	p<†
Vag. Pruritus	1.84	0.67	0.96[‡]	0.82	0.40	0.63	− 0.56	− 0.84 ↔ − 0.27	.005
Vag. Burning	1.68	0.79	0.92[‡]	0.93	0.32	0.61	− 0.60	− 0.84 ↔ − 0.35	.0005
Vag. Discharge	2.00	0.85	0.96[‡]	0.87	0.64	0.62	− 0.32	− 0.62 ↔ − 0.01	.05
VSS mean	1.83	0.78	0.95[‡]	0.88	0.45	0.64	− 0.49	− 0.64 ↔ − 0.33	.0005
Abdom. bloating	2.12	0.71	1.76	0.95	0.72	0.72	− 1.04	− 1.31 ↔ − 0.76	.0005
Abdominal pain	1.56	0.80	1.28[‡]	0.92	0.36	0.48	− 0.92	− 1.19 ↔ − 0.64	.0005
Nausea	1.76	0.71	1.56	0.90	0.52	0.57	− 1.04	− 1.27 ↔ − 0.80	.0005
Diarrhea	0.64	0.79	0.16	0.37	0.08	0.27	− 0.08	− 0.21 ↔ 0.056	ns
Constipation	1.84	0.97	1.60[‡]	0.98	0.56	0.57	− 1.04	− 1.29 ↔ − 0.78	.0005
Perianal prur's	1.44	0.70	0.68	0.84	0.24	0.43	− 0.44	− 0.72 ↔ − 0.15	.01
Menstrual irreg.	1.48	1.20	0.64	0.79	0.40	0.75	− 0.24[§]		.01
Premen. distress	2.60	0.89	1.92[‡]	1.13	0.84	0.92	− 1.08	− 1.42 ↔ − 0.73	.0005
Memory	2.04	0.77	1.84	0.92	0.76	0.65	− 1.08	− 1.35 ↔ − 0.80	.0005
Concentration	2.24	0.76	1.92	0.89	0.68	0.68	− 1.24	− 1.52 ↔ − 0.95	.0005
Depression	2.28	0.78	1.64	1.02	0.76	0.91	− 0.88	− 1.19 ↔ − 0.56	.0005

Lethargy	2.24	0.51	1.72	1.04	0.72	0.60	− 1.00	− 1.41 ↔ − 0.58	.0005
Rhinitis	2.20	1.10	1.88	1.21	0.92	0.89	− 0.96	− 1.36 ↔ − 0.55	.0005
Sneezing	0.72	0.72	0.60[‡]	0.69	0.20	0.40	− 0.40	− 0.62 ↔ − 0.17	.005
Wheezing	0.76	0.86	0.84	1.08	0.28	0.72	− 0.56	− 0.87 ↔ − 0.24	.005
NVSS mean	1.73	1.03	1.34	1.10	0.54	0.71	− 0.80	− 0.87 ↔ − 0.72	.0005
Somatization	68.88	16.28	64.92	16.73	50.58	13.41	−14.4	−17.8 ↔ −10.8	.0005
Obsess-Comp	74.62	5.62	69.46	9.85	54.65	8.51	−14.8	−17.7 ↔ −11.8	.0005
Sensitivity	71.54	6.97	64.77	12.29	51.04	10.09	−13.7	−17.0 ↔ −10.3	.0005
Depression	71.73	5.98	65.69	8.68	51.23	10.23	−14.5	−17.7 ↔ −11.1	.0005
Anxiety	72.04	8.06	65.50	9.76	52.19	9.70	−13.3	−15.8 ↔ −10.8	.0005
Hostility	71.15	6.63	64.23	11.43	52.19	9.45	−12.0	−15.0 ↔ − 9.0	.0005
Anxiety	63.77	10.40	58.65	12.88	50.96	9.42	− 7.7	−10.0 ↔ − 5.3	.0005
Ideation	62.81	11.83	58.62	12.07	46.85	7.97	−11.8	−14.5 ↔ − 8.9	.0005
Psychoticism	67.81	9.23	63.27	10.77	51.00	8.83	−12.3	−15.8 ↔ − 8.7	.0005
PSS mean	69.51	9.32	63.83	11.64	51.12	9.43	−12.7	−13.7 ↔ −11.6	.0005
Digit Span[‖]	14.45	3.64	16.09	3.03	17.56	2.82	3.4	1.0 ↔ 5.8	.05[¶]

*Week 0, preceding treatment; Week 32, end of nystatin/placebo treatment; Week 58, end of full treatment. *Confidence Interval* - Ninety-five percent interval (Mean difference, Week 32-58 ± $t_{.05}$ × Standard Error of difference). *VSS* - Mean of 3 vaginal symptoms on 0-3 scale of symptom severity; *NVSS* - Mean of 15 non-vaginal symptoms (same scale); *PSS*: Mean of 9 symptoms on SCL-90-R (standardized scales with mean of 50 and SD of 10); *Digit Span* - Scaled scores for 25-34 age group, WAIS-R.

[†] By correlated *t*-test, one-tail, df = 24.

[‡] Significant improvement, per UAB study.

[§] At Week 32, 14 of the 25 patients had no symptoms (score of 0), and eleven patients scored 1 or 2. At Week 58 seven were improved, 1 worse, and 3 unchanged. Improvement of these 11 patients was significant, P < .01, 1-tail, by correlated *t*-test.

[‖] Standard scores for 25-34 age group of WAIS-R (norm is 10).

[¶] df = 22

priately, though their case records indicated that both were asymptomatic by the fifth month of FT. Thus, our results are reported on 25 women who completed FT.

Full-Treatment Protocol

(1) Oral Nystatin: Oral nystatin was administered 4 times daily, preferably before meals, as nystatin powder suspended in water or other liquid, "swished around" in the mouth for 30-60 seconds before swallowing. After an initial dose of 2 million units (m.u.) daily, the relief of gastrointestinal symptoms determined the effective daily dose, three patients reaching 16 m.u., one patient 4 m.u., and 21 patients the same 8 m.u. maximum reached in the UAB study. Wade et al (27) used a dose of 30 m.u. daily for less sensitive strains of C. albicans.

Vaginal: Vaginal nystatin therapy consisted of the twice-daily insertion of one #4 gelatin capsule containing 500,000 units of powdered nystatin. In contrast, only one vaginal capsule was inserted daily in the UAB study.

(2) Diet: Diet minimized the intake of both yeast and carbohydrates—the former because allergic reactions to products of infectious agents (including yeast) may at times occur, the latter to reduce the amount of glucose available for fermentation by remaining viable yeast not reached by nystatin. A target was set of approximately 80 gms total sugars and starches, caloric intake being approximately 2,000-2,200/day.

(3) Immunotherapy: Immunotherapy was with C. albicans extract (Hollister-Steir) beginning with the 15th 1:10 dilution twice weekly. Thereafter increases in strength were individualized according to patients' responses as described previously (12). Inhalant allergies were diagnosed by history and skin tests and treated by standard methods, dosage and interval varying according to season, symptoms, and individual response to the injections.

(4) Avoidance: To the extent possible patients were asked to avoid antibiotics, progesterone-containing hormones, and immunosuppressant therapy to prevent the stimulation of yeast growth by these various factors.

Compliance Monitoring: Compliance of patients with the recommended treatment, monitored by the senior author at the time of office visits at 1-4 week intervals, was considered excellent, with only occasional omission of nystatin due to forgetfulness, or occasional departure from the diet.

Outcome Measures: The questionnaires used at Week 58 were those of the UAB nystatin study. Briefly, these were: (1) a symptom checklist (designed specifically for the UAB study) consisting of a four-step rating scale (0-3) of the severity of three vaginal (VS) and 15 non-vaginal (NVS) symptoms; (2) a psychological instrument, the SCL-90-R, a 90-item self-report symptom inventory that provides standardized scores on nine different psychological symptoms (PS) showing current clinical status, machine-graded by the company providing it; and (3) the digit-span (DS) test (Form III) of the Wechsler Adult Intelligence Scales-Rev. (28), used to attempt quantification of the symptom of short-term memory loss.

Design: The full- treatment research design may be characterized as a simple within-subject A-B design, comparing as baseline each patient's scores on 28 individual symptoms at the end of 32 weeks of nystatin-placebo treatment (A) to her scores at Week 58 after six months of full treatment (B).

Hypotheses: In the UAB study, the hypothesis was that some or all of these general symptoms would be reduced by nystatin. In the FT study, the hypothesis was that some or all of these general symptoms would be *further* reduced. Significant reduction of a general symptom with treatment that cleared the local symptoms of superficial yeast infection would implicate yeast as a probable cause of that general symptom.

We now report the changes in each of 28 symptoms at the end of 6-months of FT that began for each patient immediately following completion of the UAB study. Symptom scores at 32 weeks, the end of the UAB study and therefore (a conservative) baseline for the follow-up study, are compared to those at 58 weeks, the end of the FT study.

Results

Nystatin Therapy Alone

The UAB paper reported statistically significant improvement by week 32 for each of the 3 VS as well as their mean (Figs. 1, 2A, Table 1), and for four of the 25 general (NVS, PS, DS) outcome measures (Figs. 2B, 2C, Table 1). DS was reported significant, but in the "wrong" direction (data not shown in the UAB report, but see Fig. 3, Table 1). The UAB study authors concluded that nystatin was no more effective than placebo in significantly reducing general symptoms (NVS, PS, DS) described by women with chronic yeast vaginitis.

Yet on nystatin alone (Table 1) improvement occurred (as predicted) in 24 of the 25 general outcome measures. This occurred in 14 of 15 NVS (Fig. 2B), in 9 of 9 PS (Fig. 2C), and in DS (Fig. 3). By exact probability (sign test), the number of symptoms improving greatly exceeded those worsening, $P<.0000008$, allowing rejection of the null hypothesis of equal numbers of symptoms randomly becoming better or worse. Thus, in women with chronic yeast vaginitis, generalized symptoms may be caused by yeast.

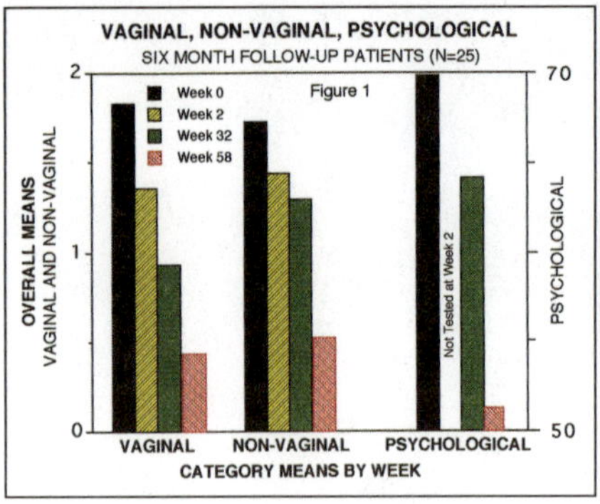

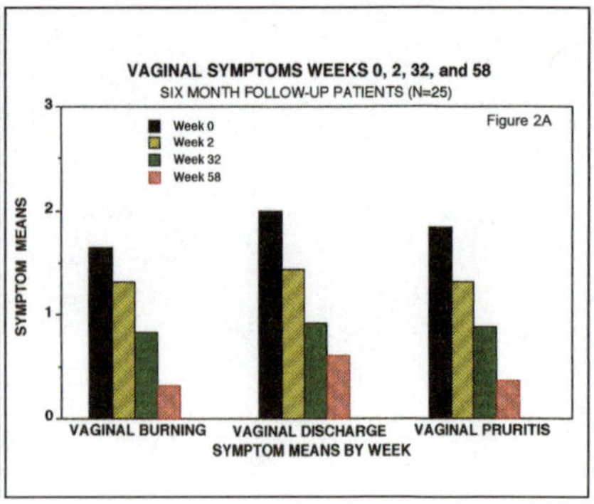

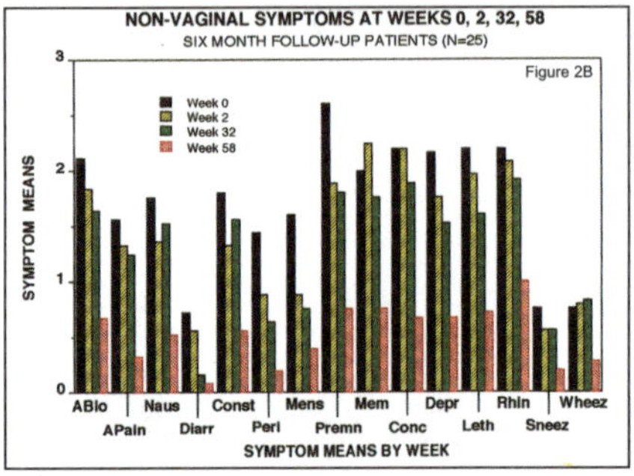

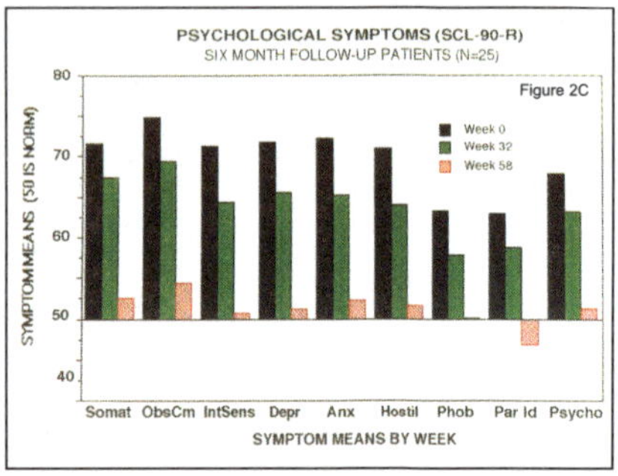

FIGURE 1 (Upper left panel). Means by symptom category for the 25 follow-up patients by key weeks. Weeks 0, 2, and 32 are drawn from the UAB study for follow-up patients only. Week 58 is the end of the full treatment. The vaginal category is the mean rating of 3 symptoms, the non-vaginal of 15 (both left vertical axis), and the psychological of 9 (right vertical axis) The psychological scale has been adjusted to make Week 0 approximately the same height as the other two scales. The psychological scale norm is 50, SD = 10. Improvements from Weeks 32 to 58 is highly significant (P < .001) for each of the 3 categories.

FIGURE 2. Means of individual symptoms for 25 follow-up patients at key weeks, grouped by category (vaginal, non-vaginal, and psychological). By one-tailed *t*-tests, significant improvement occurred in 27 of the 28 individual symptoms from Week 32 to Week 58, *(2-A)* (Upper right panel) *Vaginal* – All 3 symptoms improved, with vaginal burning, P < .001, vaginal discharge, P < .05, and vaginal pruritus, P < .005). *(2-B)* (Lower left panel) All 15 *non-vaginal* symptoms declined, with 14 of 15, P < .01 (diarrhea declined significantly, P < .01, 2-tailed, from .72 at Week 0 to .16 at Week 32, then by half gain (ns) to .08 at Week 58). *(2-C)* (Lower right panel) All 9 *psychological measures* returned to normal, each significan t at P < .001.

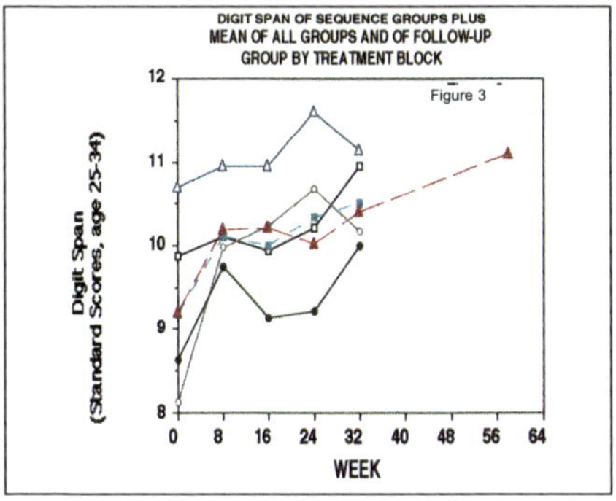

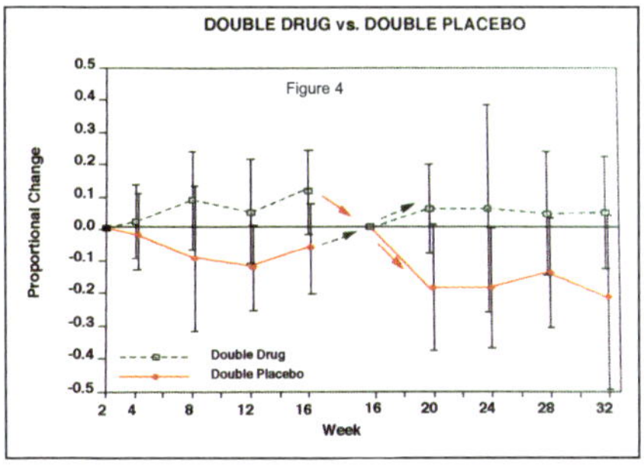

FIGURE 3. (Top panel). Mean digit spans at end of each eight-week treatment regimen for the four treatment sequence groups, Weeks 0-32. Also shown are the overall means for the 13 non-continuing patients, blue, Weeks 0-32 (Group 4), and for the 25 follow-up patients, red, Weeks 0-58. The overall mean of each of the 4 treatment groups increases from Week o to Week 32 (indiviudally, the increases are 1.3, .5, .36, and .44 digits), significant overall by paired *t*-test (P < .05, 1-tailed, 3 df). Means fro the 25 continuing and 13 non-continuing patients are shown. The size of the increase for the full treatment patients was significantly correlated with their (starting) DS at Week 32 ($r = -.71$, P < .001, df = 21). Greater improvement thus was associated with shorter initial DS. Mean DS at Week 58 was significantly greater when corrected for the (starting) level at Week 32 (P < .05, 2-tailed).

FIGURE 4. (Bottom Panel). Double Drug (green, dashed) versus Double Placebo (red, solid) groups. Adapted from UAB study Figs. 3A and 3B. UAB study patients aere grouped into double drug (16 wk total, 940 m.u.) and double placebo (16 wk. total, 11 m.u.) groups by 16-week halves of the UAB study. Treatment regimens were reversed at the start of the second 16 weeks. By Week 8 the gtoups differed in the predicted direction (positive scores indicate improvement). By Week 12 the difference nearly attained significance (P < .053, 1-tailed), and did so by Week 16 (< .03, 1-tailed). By Week 20, four weeks after the reversal in group regimens. "Double Drug" again is significantly better than "Double Placebo" (P < .05, 1-tailed). The vertical bars represent plus or minus two standard errors of the mean. Over 32 weeks "Double Drug" is significantly better than "Double Placebo," (P < .01, by ANVA).

The UAB report also compared the NVSS of patients on high-dose nystatin to the NVSS of patients on low-dose nystatin (designated "Double-drug" and "Double-placebo" respectively in the UAB report). This comparison was shown separately for each 16-week half of the study, before and after the group which was on double-drug for the first 16 weeks was switched to double-placebo, and the group on double-placebo the first 16 weeks was switched to double-drug. Each group remained on its new regimen for the final half (16 weeks) of the study (see Figs. 3A and 3B of the UAB paper and Fig. 4 herein). By ANOVA for each half of the study, significance was not found. However, in a "Letter to the Editor" (26), this comparison was shown by 4 statistical methods to be significant, favoring the group receiving "double-drug."

This comparison in two rather than the original four groups has two major advantages. It permits the use of the more powerful *t* test in a "between-subjects" comparison of the effectiveness of nystatin therapy to that of placebo, and it also increases the power of the analysis because it approximately doubles *n* (subjects per group) from 10 to 20. Using Student's *t* test, significance attained $P<.03$, 1-tail, at the end of the first half (16th week) of the UAB. study. This finding was powerfully replicated in the second half of the study when the NVSS of each group changed in the predicted (opposite) direction, $P<.05$, 1-tail, within just 4 weeks following the reversal of regimens after week 16. Also significant was a meta-analysis, $P<.015$, 2-tail, and an ANOVA, $P<.05$, over weeks 2-32 (the UAB report presented ANOVAs for weeks 2-16, and 16-32, neither of which quite reached significance, $P<.064$ and $P<.116$. It did not present an ANOVA over the full 32 weeks.)

Also, we made further analyses of the 4 original UAB treatment regimens (nystatin dose patterns) by Analysis of Covariance*, using adjusted deviation scores, controlling for several variables. Those that proved relevant included start level and block for NVSS, and start level, block, non-vaginal symptom means, and allergy season for PSS. These analyses show that there is a significant linear trend (a more powerful test than an ANOVA) in both NVSS and PSS by treatment level (Figs. 5A & 5B), $P<.03$ and $P<.01$, respectively. Thus symptoms improved progressively through the 4 treatment levels as the amount

*Myers (29) states that ". . . one should generally be interested in covariance as a technique for reducing error variance". He further states that "The concomitant data can be used after the fact if the covariance analysis is applied." He concludes ". . . data can be collected and analysis of covariance carried out even though this had not been planned before the data was collected."

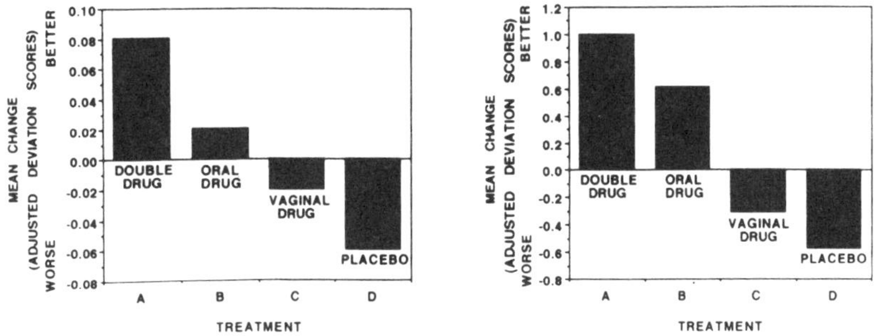

FIGURE 5 Improvement by nystatin dose during the UAB study using adjusted deviation scores (adjusted for several control variables, see text). Treatments (8 week blocks): (A) Oral and vaginal nystatin, 313.6 m.u.; (B) Oral nystatin and vaginal placebo, 308 m.u.; (C) Oral placebo and vaginal nystatin, 5.6 m.u.; (D) Oral and vaginal placebo. Dosage: Oral nystatin- Two m.u. units daily for two weeks; 4 m.u. daily for two weeks; 8 m.u. daily for four weeks. Vaginal nystatin- .1 m.u. daily for 8 weeks. *(5-A)* (Left panel) Non-vaginal symptom scores. *(5-B)* (Right panel) Psychological measures. Bars in each figure show deviations for each treatment from the overall adjusted mean of the 15 NVS, and from the overall adjusted mean of the 9 PS. Linear trend is significant, $P < .03$ and $P < .01$, respectively.

of nystatin increased step-wise from all-placebo to all-nystatin; the greater the amount of nystatin, the greater was the improvement.

From the four significant analyses reported in our "Letter to the Editor", from the 2 significant linear trend analyses, and from the finding of improvement in 24 of 25 general symptoms, it is apparent that the proposal of an etiologic role for yeast in the production of these symptoms is strongly supported by the UAB study data. The reasons why these further analyses of the UAB data showed statistically highly significant improvement with nystatin therapy, while the UAB analyses did not, are detailed in the "Discussion."

Results of Six Month Full Treatment Follow-Up Study

The six-month full treatment follow-up study reported herein shows large and highly significant further reductions in symptom severity scores in each of the 4 categories as well as for *27 of the 28* symptoms. Of the individual symptoms, only diarrhea (already near zero at week 32) is not significant. The analyses by individual patient show the impressive consistency of improvement in nearly all patients in all categories with the exception of DS, a short-term memory test, in those subjects initially scoring well above normal.

Presentation of Results

Results of outcome measures for the 25 full-treatment patients for key weeks of the UAB study, and for Week 58 after six months full treatment (weeks 32-58), are presented in three analyses:

(1) *By category* - means of the symptom scores in each category: 3 vaginal (VSS), 15 non-vaginal (NVSS), 9 psychological (PSS), digit, span (DS) (Figs. 1, 3, Table 1).

(2) *By symptom* - the average over all 25 subjects for each of the 28 outcome measures for Weeks 0, 2, 32 (extracted from the UAB data), plus Week 58 (Figs. 2A, 2B, 2C, 3, Table 1).

(3) *By patient* - for each patient, her overall average in each category, VSS, NVSS, PSS, and DS (Figs. 6A, 6B, 6C, 6D), for week 32 vs week 58. Table 2 shows these category means for individual patients for all weeks of the two studies.

Results by Category: Changes in Means of Each Symptom Category (VSS, NVSS, PSS, DS) for the Full-Treatment Patients–Week 32 to Week 58:

Mean symptom severity ratings are presented in Fig. 1 by category for VSS, NVSS, and PSS for the 25 patients at Weeks 0, 2 (not available for PSS), 32, and 58. The data are presented in Tables 1 and 2. In Fig. 1 the VSS (3 symptoms) and NVSS (15 symptoms) use the 0-3 scale on the left vertical axis. The PSS (9 scales) uses the right vertical axis. The height of the PSS scale has been adjusted so that the Week 0 bar height approximates that of the VSS and NVSS. The PS scales yield standard scores where the norm (designed average score) is 50 rather than zero. Deviations above or below 50 are departures from normal. All patients had PS scores substantially above 50 at Week 0. The PSS of the 25 subjects in the full treatment group, 69.7 at week 0, had returned to 51.2 by week 58 (Table 1), allowing the lower limit to be set at 50 in Fig. 1.

Figure 3 shows DS means for each of the 4 sequence groups of the UAB study over the first 32 weeks. It also shows DS means to week 32 for the 13 subjects who did not continue with full treatment, and DS means to week 58 for the 25 full treatment subjects (see also Tables 1, 2). Used as norms were DS for the 25-34 age group.

Symptom severity category scores for VSS, NVSS, and PSS all declined from Week 32 to Week 58, each highly significant, $P<.001$ (Ta-

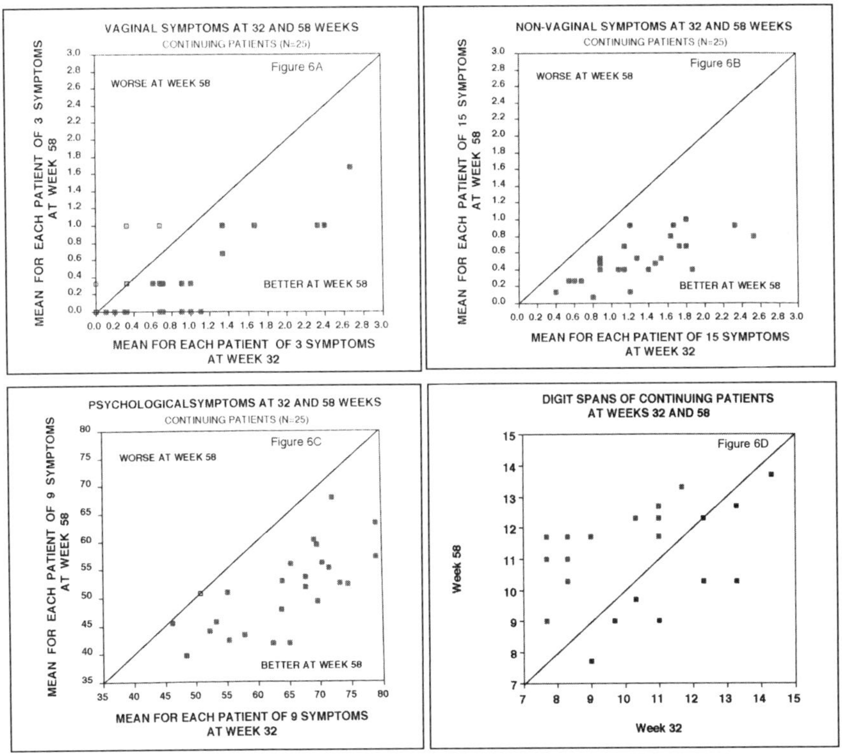

FIGURE 6. Vaginal, non-vaginal, psychological, and digit span category means of each of the 25 individual full treatment follow-up patients for Week 32 (end of UAB study and start of follow-up study) and Week 58. Each patient's score at Week 32 is read on the baseline (x-axis) and at Week 58 on the y-axis. The same score at Weeks 32 and 58 plots on the diagonal. Patients who improved (symptoms less severe) plot below the diagonal, those worse, above (except Ds), *(6-A) Vaginal* (Upper left panel) More patients, in red, improved (19) than worsened, green, (3), P < .001, 1 df (2 were at 0, and one at .33 at Week 32 and at Week 58). Amount of improvement correlates significantly with Week 32 score (*r* = .72, P < .001 2-tailed, 23 df), with higher (more severe) initial symptom scores tending strongly to result in greater improvement at Week 58. *(6-B) Non-vaginal* (Upper right panel) All 25 patients, in red, improved (P < .001, 1df). Amount of improvement is significantly correlated with Week 32 score (*r* = .70, P < .001, 2-tailed, 23 df). *(6-C) Psychological* (Lower left panel) Twenty-four patients improved, in red, and one remained the same, black (P < .001, 1 df). Amount of improvement was significantly correlated with score at Week 32 (*r* = .71, P < .001, 2-tailed, 23 df), with higher (more deviant) initial scores tending strongly to shw greater improvement at Week 58. *(6-D) Digit Span* (Lower right panel) In the DS category (the opposite of the first three categories), those whose DS improved, in red (i.e., were able to remember a longer string of digits) plot *above* the diagonal and those whose DS worsened, green, plot *belo* (see text).

TABLE 2

Mean Category Scores by Week for all Patients

		NVSS	NVSS	NVSS	NVSS	NVSS	NVSS	NVSS	NVSS	NVSS	NVSS	NVSS	PSS	PSS	PSS	PSS	PSS	PSS	VSS	VSS	VSS	VSS	VSS	VSS	VSS	VSS	VSS	VSS	VSS	DS	DS	DS	DS	DS	DS
Week		0	2	4	8	12	16	20	24	28	32	58	0	8	16	24	32	58	0	2	4	8	12	16	20	24	28	32	58	0	8	16	24	32	58
PT#	GP																																		
															SIX MONTH FOLLOW-UP GROUP																				
101	4	1.87	1.07	1.20	0.67	1.67	2.07	1.73	1.73	1.93	1.47	0.47	70.89	58.89	74.00	70.00	69.56	49.33	2.33	1.33	1.67	1.00	0.33	1.00	1.33	1.33	1.33	1.00	0.33	15	14	15	15	15	14
102	3	1.71	1.50	0.79	1.21	1.00	0.86	1.43	0.71	1.64	1.64	0.80	74.33	61.44	60.11	59.22	65.33	55.89	2.00	2.00	0.67	0.33	0.33	0.67	1.00	0.67	0.67	0.33	1.00	16	16	13	14	16	19
103	1	2.20	1.13	1.07	0.80	1.87	1.13	0.47	0.73	1.93	1.27	0.53	75.44	54.89	64.33	66.22	74.56	52.33	2.33	1.00	0.33	0.00	0.33	0.67	0.00	0.00	0.67	0.33	0.00	19	16	19	18	18	21
104	2	2.29	2.20	2.13	2.13	1.60	1.73	1.80	1.13	1.80	2.33	0.93	70.89	66.56	68.00	61.22	73.22	52.56	1.67	1.00	1.00	1.00	0.67	1.67	0.00	0.00	0.00	0.67	0.33	16	19	14	21	13	18
106	1	1.87	1.47	1.13	1.00	0.73	0.80	1.93	1.07	0.87	1.87	0.40	68.89	58.11	51.44	51.11	53.22	42.44	2.00	1.00	0.33	1.33	0.33	0.00	1.00	0.67	0.33	1.00	0.33	15	17	17	15	17	18
108	4	1.60	1.67	1.33	0.93	1.20	1.13	1.27	1.07	1.00	1.20	0.13	77.89	67.56	68.22	64.11	67.78	51.89	2.00	1.67	0.67	1.00	1.00	1.00	1.00	1.00	0.67	1.00	0.00	15	12	15	11	12	14
109	1	1.87	1.87	1.33	1.47	1.80	1.73	1.07	1.20	0.87	1.07	0.40	76.11	70.67	79.11	67.11	65.11	41.89	1.33	1.67	0.00	0.00	0.33	1.33	1.67	0.00	0.00	0.00	0.00	14	13	13	15	16	15
113	1	2.07	2.13	1.93	1.80	1.47	1.40	1.87	2.13	0.60	0.60	0.27	62.78	58.89	52.00	66.22	46.22	45.56	2.00	2.00	2.00	1.67	1.00	1.00	1.33	1.67	0.67	0.00	0.00	13	15	14	15	17	14
114	3	2.07	1.93	1.53	1.53	0.60	0.53	0.73	1.27	0.53	1.53	0.53	63.44	61.00	45.00	58.44	57.78	43.33	1.67	1.00	1.00	1.00	0.67	0.33	0.67	0.67	0.00	1.00	0.00	20	19	20	18	21	16
115	2	1.57	1.27	1.53	0.80	1.07	1.27	1.47	1.13	1.73	1.13	0.67	63.78	50.44	61.33	57.00	53.33	45.67	1.33	2.00	1.00	0.00	0.67	0.67	0.33	0.00	0.00	0.00	0.33						24
118	1	1.00	1.20	1.53	1.33	0.93	1.00	0.93	0.93	1.00	0.67	0.27	63.44	57.78	58.00	55.67	50.67	50.78	2.00	1.00	1.00	0.67	1.00	1.00	1.67	2.33	1.33	1.33	1.00	15	20	17	19	14	18
123	1	2.13	1.87	1.40	1.87	1.40	1.47	1.53	2.27	1.27	1.20	0.93	77.11	76.44	77.67	79.89	72.11	67.89	2.00	1.33	1.67	1.00	1.67	1.33	1.00	2.00	1.67	0.67	0.33	17	18	17	18	17	20
125	3	1.60	0.73	1.00	1.27	0.87	1.07	1.00	1.40	0.47	0.87	0.40	62.00	64.89	65.67	62.56	64.00	52.89	3.00	2.00	2.67	3.00	3.00	2.00	3.00	1.67	2.67	2.67	1.67	6	13	17	15	17	14

129	4	1.60	1.33	1.13	1.27	1.07	0.93	0.87	0.53	1.00	1.13	0.40	63.78	62.33	62.22	50.44	62.33	41.78	0.00	0.00	0.00	0.33	0.00	0.00	0.00	0.33	0.00	0.33	0.33	6	11	13	13	14	12
130	2	1.36	0.53	0.87	0.27	0.53	1.00	0.73	0.07	1.07	0.53	0.27	68.22	49.22	51.67	42.44	52.11	44.11	2.00	0.67	0.00	0.00	0.33	3.00	0.33	0.00	0.33	0.67	0.00	13	17	17	13	13	16
131	3	1.80	0.80	1.20	1.60	1.33	1.40	1.13	0.80	1.40	0.87	0.47	74.56	69.78	68.00	60.89	70.33	56.11	2.00	1.33	0.67	1.00	0.33	0.33	1.00	0.67	1.00	0.67	0.00	12	14	16	15	12	18
136	1	2.33	2.07	2.00	2.27	1.87	2.27	2.47	2.00	2.33	2.53	0.80	80.22	80.44	81.00	70.33	79.00	57.22	2.67	2.00	1.67	2.67	1.67	1.67	2.00	1.67	2.00	2.33	1.00	11	14	9	9	12	17
137	4	1.67	0.93	1.13	1.07	1.07	0.80	1.27	1.20	1.20	1.40	0.40	66.00	63.67	55.78	57.67	63.78	47.89	1.67	2.00	1.67	1.33	0.33	0.67	0.33	0.67	0.67	0.67	0.33	15	18	17	11	17	20
139	2	1.07	1.00	0.93	0.87	1.13	1.13	0.87	0.93	1.07	0.87	0.53	62.22	56.78	57.89	54.89	55.11	50.89	1.67	1.33	1.33	0.67	1.00	0.67	0.67	1.00	1.67	0.67	1.00	21	20	21	20	23	22
141	1	1.93	1.80	1.87	1.53	1.67	1.33	1.40	1.33	1.47	1.67	0.93	76.78	73.78	72.22	70.44	71.56	55.33	1.00	1.00	2.67	1.00	0.33	0.33	0.67	0.67	0.00	1.33	0.67						17
143	3	1.33	1.40	1.53	1.20	1.27	1.27	1.60	1.73	1.40	1.80	1.00	68.44	62.78	67.00	75.56	69.22	60.22	2.00	2.00	2.00	1.67	1.33	2.00	1.67	2.00	2.00	2.33	1.00						20
145	3	2.07	1.00	0.93	1.00	1.87	1.53	1.47	2.00	2.00	1.80	0.67	80.44	75.00	80.00	81.00	79.11	63.44	2.67	2.67	1.67	1.33	2.00	1.67	2.00	2.00	2.00	1.67	1.00	12	14	13	14	13	17
147	4	1.07	0.93	1.13	1.13	1.27	0.87	1.20	1.00	0.80	0.80	0.07	54.78	51.67	49.78	49.89	48.44	39.67	1.00	1.00	1.00	1.33	0.67	0.33	1.00	1.00	1.00	1.00	0.00	14	15	13	13	17	19
149	1	1.80	1.93	1.73	1.00	1.80	1.93	1.67	0.87	1.80	1.73	0.67	67.22	61.56	69.22	60.44	67.67	53.67	1.67	1.00	0.67	0.33	0.33	0.67	0.00	0.67	0.67	0.33	0.00	18	16	22	19	21	20
107	3	1.53	1.13	1.10	1.00	1.23	1.20	1.47	1.60	1.07	1.53	0.46	74.22	67.11	63.11	71.33	69.70	59.33	2.00	1.00	0.67	1.33	0.67	0.33	1.33	3.00	1.00	1.67	0.67	15	16	18	23	19	16
MEAN		1.74	1.40	1.34	1.24	1.29	1.27	1.34	1.23	1.29	1.34	0.53	69.75	63.26	64.11	62.56	64.05	51.28	1.84	1.40	1.12	1.00	0.81	0.97	1.00	1.03	0.89	0.95	0.45	14.5	15.8	15.9	15.6	16.1	17.6

SIX MONTH FOLLOW-UP PATIENTS WITH INCOMPLETE DATA

117	4	1.47	1.60	1.67	1.60	1.27	1.47	0.40	0.33	0.47	0.40	0.13	46.44	48.11	52.00	39.67	37.00	NA*	1.67	0.00	1.67	2.67	0.33	0.00	1.00	1.67	0.00	0.00	NA	14	17	16	15	19	19

TABLE 2 (continued)

142	2	1.14	1.13	0.93	1.47	1.33	1.07	0.87	0.87	0.87	1.13	NA	71.78	70.22	63.78	65.89	64.89	NA	2.00	2.33	1.00	2.33	2.00	1.33	0.67	1.00	2.00	1.33	NA						
MEAN		1.70	1.39	1.34	1.26	1.29	1.27	1.28	1.19	1.24	1.30		68.96	62.96	63.65	61.83	63.07		1.84	1.38	1.14	1.11	0.84	0.95	0.99	1.05	0.90	0.93	0.42	14.4	15.8	15.9	15.6	16.2	17.6
THIRTY-TWO WEEKS ONLY GROUP																																			
110	3	1.20	0.73	0.33	0.27	0.60	0.47	0.60	0.80	0.93	0.73		63.78	58.11	52.67	52.00	48.67		1.33	0.67	1.00	0.33	0.00	0.33	0.33	0.33	0.00	0.33		14	15	15	20	16	
112	4	1.40	1.07	0.93	1.13	1.60	0.87	1.27	0.93	1.07	0.67		74.33	67.56	62.89	73.89	63.67		1.67	2.33	2.33	2.33	0.00	0.00	0.67	0.33	0.00	0.00		19	18	16	20	20	
119	3	2.33	1.73	2.47	1.87	1.27	1.13	1.93	2.07	1.87	2.07		70.22	78.89	74.56	78.44	68.22		2.00	2.33	2.33	2.00	0.33	1.00	2.33	2.33	2.00	1.33		6	9	13	9	13	
120	2	1.36	0.67	0.33	1.40	0.80	0.53	0.40	1.60	0.80	0.80		71.00	71.89	57.33	62.78	54.11		2.00	1.67	0.00	0.00	0.33	0.00	0.67	1.33	1.00	1.00		16	14	15	17	16	
121	2	1.86	0.80	1.27	1.07	0.93	1.07	1.20	1.20	0.67	0.93		72.22	64.89	51.89	55.78	54.44		2.00	1.00	1.67	2.00	2.00	0.67	1.67	1.00	0.33	1.33		16	14	17	17	19	
122	3	1.60	1.53	1.33	2.00	1.47	1.67	1.27	1.87	1.20	1.60		69.00	76.67	67.44	77.33	68.11		2.00	1.00	1.00	2.33	1.67	1.33	1.33	1.33	2.33	1.67		14	18	19	19	17	
124	4	2.27	2.00	2.00	1.53	2.53	2.67	2.27	1.27	2.53	2.47		73.78	68.22	76.33	64.00	73.22		1.67	1.33	1.67	2.00	2.33	2.00	1.33	1.67	1.00	1.00		12	13	9	11	9	
135	3	1.60	1.13	1.73	0.07	1.67	0.47	1.73	0.60	1.73	1.07		55.44	51.78	46.22	50.89	54.33		1.33	0.33	0.33	0.00	0.00	1.00	0.00	0.67	0.00	0.00		14	18	14	19	12	
138	3	1.87	1.21	1.29	1.67	0.64	1.13	0.86	1.47	0.71	0.73		72.22	73.89	65.11	66.78	66.67		1.00	1.67	0.33	0.00	0.00	0.00	0.67	0.67	0.00	0.00		13	18	17	17	18	
140	1	2.60	2.07	2.00	2.00	1.53	1.67	1.33	1.60	2.27	0.93		80.33	78.33	76.89	77.56	68.89		2.67	2.67	2.67	2.00	2.00	1.67	2.00	2.67	2.00	1.33		15	14	11	14	18	
146	1	1.80	1.33	1.33	1.00	1.13	1.13	1.40	1.13	1.40	1.33		64.11	57.44	57.22	55.33	56.78		1.67	0.67	0.00	0.00	0.67	0.67	0.33	1.00	0.33	0.67		16	14	16	16	20	
148	2	1.79	1.27	0.93	2.07	1.27	1.67	0.73	1.67	0.67	1.40		73.56	72.00	64.78	71.56	70.00		1.67	2.00	2.00	2.33	2.67	2.00	1.00	1.00	1.67	1.00		18	18	18	21	21	
150	4	1.67	1.20	1.07	1.27	1.40	1.20	0.93	1.20	1.27	1.07		65.44	64.33	61.22	57.33	59.56		1.67	0.67	1.00	0.67	0.67	2.00	0.67	1.33	0.67	1.00		12	18	14	21	17	
MEAN		1.79	1.29	1.31	1.33	1.30	1.21	1.22	1.34	1.32	1.22		69.65	68.00	62.66	64.90	62.05		1.74	1.41	1.26	1.23	0.97	0.97	1.00	1.21	0.87	0.82		14.2	15.5	14.9	17.0	16.6	

DID NOT COMPLETE 32 WEEKS

111	2	1.57	1.47	1.87	1.40	2.20	1.13	1.67	1.67	2.00	1.67	0.67	1.67
133	4	1.27	0.80	0.47	1.27			1.00	0.00	0.00	0.00		
105	2	2.00	0.47	0.47				2.00	0.33	0.33			
132	1	1.93	1.80	2.07				2.00	1.00	2.00			
144	4	1.07	0.93	1.07				1.67	2.33	0.00			
116	4	1.73	1.93					2.00	1.33				
126	1	1.40						1.00					
127	4	1.47						2.33					
128	2	1.50						1.00					
134	2	1.86						2.00					
151	2	1.57						1.33					

**Six month follow-up patients with incomplete data* - These two patients completed 6 months of full treatment. Six month PSS questionnaires of patient 117 were unusable; patient 142 did not complete the questionnaires at Week 58.

NVSS - Mean of 15 non-vaginal symptom scores (0-3 scale). *VSS* - Mean of 3 vaginal symptoms (same scale). *PSS* - Mean of 9 symptoms on SCL-90-R (standardized scales with mean of 50 and SD of 10). *DS* - Digit span (standardized scores for 25-34 age group, WAIS-R. *Week* - Weeks at which questionnaires and digit span test were completed. Week 0, preceding treatment; Weeks 2-32, UAB study, patients on one of four 8 week nystatin/placebo regimens; Week 58, at end of 26 weeks of full treatment. *GP* - Treatment group, first 32 weeks. *Six month follow-up group* - The 25 patients who completed an additional 26 weeks on full treatment. *Thirty-two weeks only group* - The 13 patients who did not continue immediately with full treatment. *Did not complete 32 weeks* - The 11 patients who dropped out of the UAB study during the first 32 weeks.

ble 1). The increase (*improvement*) in DS also was significant, P<.05, (Table 1), by analysis of variance, controlling for start level.

By Individual Symptoms: Changes in Means of Each Symptom for the 25 Full Treatment Patients–Week 32 to Week 58:

Figs. 2A, 2B, 2C (VS, NVS, PS), Fig. 3(DS), and Table 1 show that all 28 individual symptoms changed in the predicted direction from Week 32 to Week 58, with 27 significant. Twenty-five of the primary symptoms (VS, NVS and PS) reached P<.01 or P<.001. Vaginal discharge and DS reached P<.05. The one non-significant primary NV symptom (diarrhea) had decreased from .72 at Week 0, and from .56 at Week 2 to .16 at week 32, P<.01 and P<.05, yet it still decreased another 50% to .08 at Week 58 (ns).

By Individual Patient: Changes in Category Average of Individual Patients:

Table 2 and Figures 6A, 6B, 6C and 6D show the impressive consistency of improvement across patients (except DS), based on their four category averages. By Chi Square, the difference in the number of patients improving or worsening was significant in each case except DS (for which see below).

Interpretation of the Individual Patient Plots: In Figs. 6A, 6B, and 6C, note that a patient who had the same score at Week 32 and Week 58 (i.e., one whose score did not change) would plot *on* the diagonal line. One with a lower (improved) symptom score at Week 58 would plot *below* the diagonal line, while one who became *worse* would plot *above* the diagonal line. Thus a patient scoring 1.0 at Week 32 (horizontal axis), who decreases to .5 at Week 58 (vertical axis), plots below the diagonal, while one scoring .5 at Week 32 and 1.0 at Week 58 (i.e., became worse) plots above.

In contrast to vaginal, non-vaginal, and psychological symptoms, an *increase* in DS (Fig. 3, 6D) denotes *improved* short-term memory. The improved patients—those who recalled more digits at Week 58 than at Week 32—plot *above* (not below) the diagonal line (Fig. 6D), and those whose short-term memory is worse at Week 58 plot *below* the diagonal (the opposite of VSS, NVSS, PS).

VSS: Fig. 6A and Table 2 show the mean of 3 VS for each patient at Week 32 and Week 58; 19 patients improved, two were unchanged at zero, one at .33, and three were worse at Week 58. The null hypothesis (i.e., that equal numbers of patients worsened and improved) is rejected. For those changing, the Chi Square is 11.1, P<.001, df=1, with Yate's correction. Further, the amount of improvement is highly and significantly correlated with the size of each patient's initial (Week 32) score (*r* = .72, df=23, P<.001). Higher (more severe symptoms) initial scores tended strongly to result in greater reduction of VSS by Week 58.

NVSS: Fig. 6B and Table 2 show the mean of 15 NVS for each patient. All 25 patients improved from Week 32 to Week 58, with Chi Square of 23, P<<.001, df=1, with Yate's correction, allowing rejection of the null hypothesis. Again, those with the highest initial symptom severity scores tended strongly to improve the most (*r* = .70, df=23, P<.001).

PSS: Fig. 6C and Table 2 show for each patient the mean of nine PS scales from the SCL-90-R, a published and validated instrument. Twenty-four patients improved, Week 32 to Week 58, while one (already at the norm at week 32) remained unchanged, again allowing rejection of the null hypothesis, Chi Square = 22, P<<.001, df=1, with Yate's correction. Once again, the amount of improvement is highly and significantly correlated with the size of each patient's initial (Week 32) score (*r* = .71, df=23, P<.001).

DS: The DS mean for the full treatment patients at Week 58 (Fig. 3, Table 1) is significantly longer (*improved*) than their mean at Week 32, P<.05 (after correction for start level), but it can be seen (Fig. 6D) that there was much more variability among patients for this measure. The Chi Square comparing all patients who improved with those who worsened showed the numbers not to be significantly different. However, no patient improved who scored above 12 (n = 5) at Week 32 (well above the norm of 10 for this age group), while of those 18 patients initially at 12 or less, 13 improved and 5 worsened. The amount of change among all patients was significantly correlated with the DS at Week 32, with lower Week 32 scores tending strongly to result in increased digit span (i.e., *improvement* in memory) at Week 58 (*r* = .71, P<.001, df=21).

DS Versus the NV Symptoms of "Memory Loss" and "Decreased Concentration": Patients' self-rating (on the 0-3 scale) of two of the NV symptoms, "memory loss" and "concentration impairment," logically might be measuring much the same entity as DS. Memory and concentration are themselves highly correlated with each other at Weeks 32 and 58, respectively, so that there is much in common that they measure ($r = .84$ and $r = .66$ respectively, $P<.01$, for each).

However, at Week 58 neither "memory loss" nor "concentration impairment" correlates above .08 (ns) with DS. At Week 32 the corresponding correlations were $r = .43$ (18% shared variance), $P<.05$, and $r = .28$, ns. Thus, DS is largely but perhaps not entirely a measure of a different entity than either "memory loss" or "concentration impairment" as quantified by the patients on the 0-3 scale used to rate the severity of the fifteen NVS.

Discussion

It is important to note that the comparison of nystatin to placebo was carried out at UAB. The senior author of this paper selected the subjects, suggested the relevant NVS, and participated in the planning of that study but not in its execution. Patient selection was based on the presence of generalized symptoms described by women with chronic yeast vaginitis. The relationship of these NVS to the chronic yeast infections was evaluated by independent researchers in the nystatin/placebo study.

Nystatin Only

As expected in view of the accepted efficacy of nystatin in the treatment of yeast vaginitis, in the UAB study each of the 3 vaginal symptoms responded to nystatin therapy, $P<.001$. At the same time, improvement in 4 of the 25 general measures also attained significance $P<.05$ (25), but overall significance was not reported for reasons discussed below.

Why did our further analyses of the UAB study data yield statistically significant differences in non-vaginal outcome measures by nystatin dosage level when the original UAB analyses in general did not do so? The answer lies in the use of more powerful statistical methods. (This does not violate the injunction against *post hoc* testing of additional comparisons not specified in advance.) These methods still test the *a priori* hypothesis that treatment with oral and vaginal nystatin is superior to oral and vaginal placebo in reducing non-vaginal symptoms in women with diagnosed yeast vaginitis*.

*See also footnote, page 150.

In designing the UAB study, we included only enough patients in each of its four sequence groups to detect a relatively large drug effect (about one standard deviation), when in fact the size of this effect proved to be much smaller. By considering data in two rather than four groups, thus doubling the number in each group (high vs low-dose nystatin), and allowing analysis by Student's *t* test (far more powerful than the ANOVA used), significance was found at the end of the first 16 weeks and at the end of the second 16 weeks after the two groups reversed regimens, and for the 32 weeks overall.

The power of the ANOVA to detect a true effect in the Latin-Square design used computes to be less than 20%, given the number of subjects, the observed effect size, and the variability among patients. This means that it will yield significance for an effect of the size that actually occurred only about 20% of the time, while 80% of the time mistakenly indicating that treatment was without effect (false acceptance of the null hypothesis that treatment was without effect, Type II error). On the other hand, the computed power of the *t*-test for the 2 group analysis (described below) was greater than 98%, signifying that it had a greater than 98% chance of yielding significance. Under the two group comparison, the power of the ANOVA improved but was still less than 50%.

Further, it was assumed in the design of the study that there would be no carryover of effect from regimen block to regimen block. Substantial carryover did in fact occur. While the ANOVA also was run correcting for starting level of each sequence group at the beginning of each new regimen, this corrects only for linear effects, leaving non-linear carryover effects uncorrected. These effects reduce the power of the ANOVA.

Because of such carry-over effect, designs are inappropriate in which each subject serves as own control (within-subjects design). When, as with antimicrobal drugs, treatment partially or completely eradicates the etiologic agent, drug may appear no more *effective* than placebo. As an example, 10 days of penicillin therapy for an acute streptococcal sore throat usually will eradicate the streptococcus. Symptoms will be absent and will remain so through the following placebo period. Even if not eradicated, suppression of the microorganism that persists until the end of the placebo period will prevent symptoms from rebounding fully, i.e., carry-over effect.

In summary, in the UAB study partial treatment with nystatin/placebo alone, without recommended diet or immunotherapy, resulted in highly significant improvement as measured in this independently done blinded study, NVSS, PSS and DS each changing in the predicted direction (Table 2). It is also important to note that, at completion of the UAB study, each of the 27 women who immediately began full treatment stated to the senior author of this paper that the nystatin/placebo therapy had resulted in improvement in both the vaginal and generalized symptoms*. Thus, the improvement in 24 of 25 general symptoms was clinically relevant as well as statistically significant.

Full-Treatment

Following 6 months of full-treatment, as reflected in the questionnaires and digit-span test completed at Week 58 (Table 1, 2, Figs. 1 2A, 2B, 2C, 3, 5A 5B, 6A, 6B, 6C, 6D), it is apparent that these 25 women were essentially well from the multiple chronic symptoms present at week 0, which had improved but were still present at Week 32. This striking improvement on full-treatment, following the more modest improvement in 27 of 28 symptoms on nystatin alone, strongly suggests that both treatments reached the common factor underlying the local as well as the numerous, severe generalized complaints of these women. Thus, treatment attacked the *cause* of the chronic illness. The striking superiority of full treatment over nystatin alone is evident. This quantitatively important *further* reduction in symptoms was significant in all four symptom categories and for each symptom except one, thereby strongly validating the connection between yeast and these general symptoms.

The full-treatment regimen involved four substantive changes in therapy: (1) In the UAB study it had been necessary to encapsulate the oral nystatin in order to blind the taste. On full treatment, nystatin in liquid form allowed suppression of additional yeast in the mouth and esophagus, by-passed by the oral capsules used in the UAB study. Also, the dose of oral nystatin was increased as needed to control each patient's symptoms, and nystatin was administered vaginally twice rather than once daily. Once the effective daily dose was determined from symptom response, this was maintained for the remainder of the 6 months of full treatment. In contrast, in the UAB study nystatin/placebo combinations were changed every 8 weeks. (2) Diet (not controlled in the UAB study) reduced the intake of carbohydrate to minimize glucose available for fermentation by any remain-

*The fact that altogether 39 of the 40 did come for full treatment supports these opinions.

ing viable yeast, and also minimized the amount of ingested yeast in the event of hypersensitivity to yeast. (3) Immunotherapy (not employed in the UAB study)—Immunotherapy included C. albicans extract as well as inhalant antigens as indicated by history and skin tests. (4) Finally, as in the UAB study, to the extent possible therapies were avoided that stimulate yeast growth in the body (e.g., antibiotics, steroids, progesterone).

It is important to note that vaginal category means (VSS, Fig. 1) were reduced (significantly) by "full-treatment" despite having improved (also significantly) on nystatin alone in the UAB study, $P<.001$ (25). In fact, each of the three VS means showed further statistically significant decreases on full treatment, suggesting an added benefit of oral nystatin, the twice rather than once daily vaginal nystatin, and diet and immunotherapy, even when dealing with vaginal symptoms.

It was essential that it be demonstrated that these 25 patients were not significantly different from the 13 who did not continue immediately (12 of the 13 did in fact return for full treatment but at a later date). This was done by comparisons of mean scores of the two groups during the UAB study, shown in Figs. 3, 7A, 7B & 7C and in Table 2. Student's t tests of the differences in the two groups at week 32 for VSS, NVSS, PSS, and DS did not approach significance, showing that the groups did not differ. The means of the two groups in all three symptom categories and for DS, by week of testing, are provided in Table 2. Table 2 also shows data for dropouts from the UAB study, and for the 2 excluded follow-up patients.

The evidence is convincing that both nystatin and full treatment were specific for the cause of the illness, and that the efficacy of full treatment is much superior to that of nystatin alone.

Alternate Interpretations of Results

Spontaneous Remission. For spontaneous remission to have been responsible for this striking improvement, it would be necessary to assume that it occurred in 25 of 25 women for every symptom in all four categories, and that it lasted for 14 months, increasing sharply on full treatment. While theoretically possible, it is illogical to invoke spontaneous remission as an explanation for the simultaneous improvement in all symptoms and in all 25 patients.

Placebo effect. One characteristic of placebo effect is its short duration. The likelihood of a 58-week placebo effect is remote, as is the likeli-

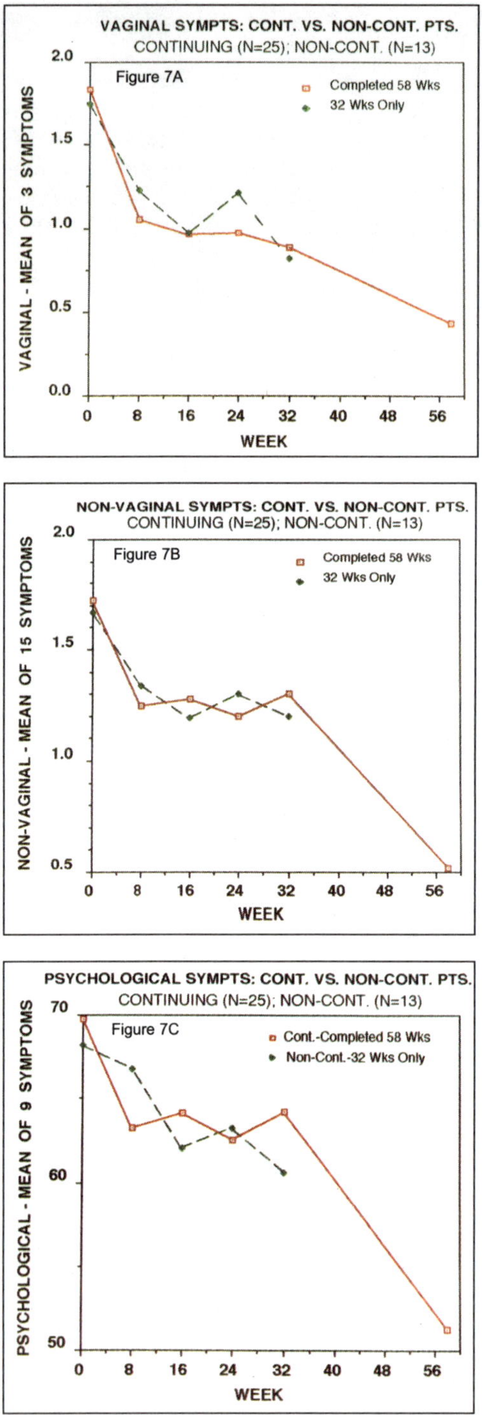

FIGURE 7
Comparison of non-continuing (N = 13) and continuing (follow-up) patients (N = 25) at the end of 8-week treatment blocks in the UAB study, plus Week 58 for continuing patients. Means are by symptom category (vaginal, non-vaginal, psychological). The groups were not significantly different over the first 32 weeks in any category. *(7-A)* (Top panel) VSS; *(7-B)* (Middle panel) NVSS; *(7-C)* (Lower panel) PSS; the corresponding DS means are shown in Figure 3.

hood of the onset of a second stronger placebo effect starting at Week 32 and lasting until week 58. This is particularly true in that, according to their medical histories, these women had failed to recover (i.e., show placebo effect!) on the many treatments received prior to the UAB study.

The brief duration of placebo effect was, in fact, noted in the UAB report. It was pointed out that all four sequence groups improved in the first two weeks (placebo effect) with no significant difference between treatment and placebo groups, but that over the remaining 6 weeks of the first treatment block, only the double-drug group continued to improve. Fig. 4 herein shows that the NVSS of the group on double placebo became and remained worse from Week 2 through week 16, while the NVSS of the group on "double drug" remained improved through week 16.

Indeed, as may be seen by inspection of Fig. 4, designated "Double-drug vs Double-placebo", in both the first and last 16 weeks, NVSS in the group on double placebo increased (became more severe). This pattern occurred not only from week 2 to week 8, but again after Week 16 as the former "double-drug" group became the "double placebo" group (also Fig. 1 (26) and Fig. 4 herein). Further, this reversal of regimens at Week 16 (blinded) was followed *immediately* by significant *improvement* in NVSS in those women now on double drug (on double placebo until Week 16). These changes in each group occurred by Week 20, only 4 weeks after this reversal, each in the direction predicted by its new regimen.

These results do not permit a "placebo effect" interpretation except during the first two weeks. In a double-blind study, placebo effect cannot shift scores in opposite directions, as occurred after regimen reversal at Week 16.

Chronic Candidiasis–a Fungus Infection, not an Allergy! In the UAB report reference was made to the "position paper" of the American Academy of Allergy (4), which stated that *allergic* reactions to C. albicans would not account for the many symptoms reported—an opinion in agreement with that of the senior author of this paper, who has consistently proposed that *toxic* (as well as possible allergic) mechanisms were responsible for the non-mucosal, general symptoms. In this position paper the term "candidiasis hypersensitivity syndrome" was coined to denote allergic manifestation to C. albicans. A recent excellent review is available concerning the possibility of allergic reactions to both protein and polysaccaride antigens of C. albicans, including immediate and delayed types, the "id" reaction, and possible Arthus-type reactions (5). Also, a recent excellent review discusses the possibility of an allergic component in the pathogenesis of yeast vaginitis (30).

It is essential to keep in mind that "chronic candidiasis" refers, not to an "allergy", but to a fungal *infection*. As with other infectious agents, there are occasions when allergic reactions do occur, as in the acute urticaria that may accompany a viral infection, and acute rheumatic fever or acute glomerulonephritis that may complicate beta-hemolytic streptococcal infections. Nevertheless, in these instances one is still dealing with infections that are named, not for the allergic manifestation that may or may not occur, but for the causative organism. Streptococcal infections are not called "streptococcal hypersensitivity syndrome" because allergic reactions to products of the microorganism do occasionally occur. The term "candidiasis hypersensitivity syndrome" is appropriate only when discussing possible hypersensitivity responses to yeast products. "Chronic candidiasis" (superficial or deep) identifies the disease by its etiologic agent.

Nevertheless, because patients with the superficial candidiasis syndrome frequently also have developed multiple food and inhalant sensitivities, as well as intolerance to environmental chemicals, it is the opinion of the senior author of this paper that consultation with an allergist often is appropriate, particularly for the more advanced cases that may require immunotherapy. Determining other allergens requiring treatment can be difficult. Elimination of offending allergens, and immunotherapy for those that cannot be avoided, remain important measures in therapy of these patients.

Yeast and the Chronic Fatigue Syndrome. The "chronic fatigue syndrome" was defined in 1988 in a report issued jointly by a number of major medical institutions (31). The symptoms reported closely parallel (Table 3) those described earlier (1978) in the superficial candidiasis syndrome (2,16)—symptoms relieved by nystatin, diet and immunotherapy. Additional indication for an etiological role for yeast in this symptom-complex was the reported (32) clearing of these symptoms with ketoconazole therapy in 84% of 1100 patients selected by the criteria set forth in the initial "chronic fatigue syndrome" paper. Lending objectivity to these results (not blinded) was the fact that 685 of the 1100 patients were on disability prior to treatment, with only 12 remaining on disability after several months of ketoconazole therapy. It was concluded that C. albicans was the cause of these symptoms "in a great majority of cases". The added therapeutic

TABLE 3

Comparison of the General Symptoms of the Superficial Candidiasis Syndrome (2,16) with Symptoms of the Chronic Fatigue Syndrome (30)

*SUPERFICIAL CANDIDIASIS SYNDROME**	*CHRONIC FATIGUE SYNDROME†*
General symptoms:	*Symptoms:*
Fatigue or lethargy	Fatigue-generalized muscle weakness
Memory loss - poor concentration	Memory and concentration impairment
Depression, anxiety	Depression, irritability
Chronic sore throat	Sore throat, pharyngitis (non-exudative)
Low-grade (only) fever	Mild fever
Insomnia	Sleep disturbances (insomnia, hypersomnia)
Cervical node enlargement (minimal)	Lymph nodes-palpable or tender cervical and axillary
Headaches	Headache-generalized
Muscle and joint pains	Myalgia and arthralgias
Hormone problems-decreased libido, acne, PMS, menstrual bleeding abnormalities	
Chemical intolerance-odors, foods, drugs	
Allergies (hives, migraine headaches, asthma, allergic rhinitis)	

*First described 1978[2], and 1986[16]
†Described 1988[29]

benefit of a low-carbohydrate diet was stressed (Jessop C., Personal communication: July 16, 1989). One important result of the defining of this syndrome was to give legitimacy to these multiple complaints by patients who heretofore had so often been dismissed as psychoneurotics.

Diagnosis of Superficial Candidiasis Syndrome. "Deep candidiasis" (systemic candidiasis) denotes yeast infections of one or more of the internal organs. It and superficial candidiasis, even though caused by the same organism, might well be thought of as two unrelated diseases, so much do they differ in seriousness, symptomatology, and in diagnosis. Once the skin/mucosal barrier is breached and yeast is seeded into the kidney, heart, brain, etc., the danger to life is real, the diagnosis difficult, and symptoms very different. Just as physicians in such specialities as gynecology, dermatology and allergy rarely see patients with deep candidiasis, it is doubtful that academic mycologists often are involved in the long-term effort to help patients with chronic, symptomatic superficial yeast infections best exemplified by women who suffer for years with yeast vaginitis—who so often ultimately are told "you will just have to learn to live with it." The existence of these two widely differing forms of chronic candidiasis—deep and superficial—and their treatment by physicians in such diverse specialities, perhaps contributes to the difficulty in mutual understanding of the varied symptoms that may be induced by yeast in these two widely divergent clinical entities.

Defining the Superficial Candidiasis Syndrome. The editorial (33) that accompanied the UAB nystatin paper commented on the difficulty of defining the reported syndrome (superficial candidiasis syndrome), citing this as an obstacle to research on this condition. This is a valid point, since it is true that a number of seemingly unrelated symptoms do occur. But a pattern may be seen that does allow accurate definition of this condition (16).

It begins with the familiar "local" symptoms at the sites of infections where yeast lives normally—the discharge, itching and burning of vaginal yeast infections; coated tongue and irritation of oral thrush; indigestion, dysphagia, and nausea of upper GI yeast infections; and the constipation and/or diarrhea, excess gas and bloating, and rectal itching of lower GI tract superficial candidisis. Often accompanying these mucosal infections are external infections under nails, between the toes or thighs, and under pendulous breasts—in short, where conditions of warmth and moisture prevail. These "local" symptoms occur in various combinations; those present at a given time in a particular patient depend upon the site or sites of skin or mucous membranes that Candida albicans has succeeded in colonizing. The first step in diagnosis is to establish that there is indeed present yeast infection of the external or internal surfaces where yeast exists as a member of the normal flora.

Thereafter the search is for the "non-local" or "general" symptoms that may appear, presumably when the yeast load has progressed to a critical point. These symptoms may be considered in several distinct categories (16): (1) lack of energy (fatigue, lethary) (2) central nervous system symptoms (inappropriate depression, anxiety, panic attacks, insomnia, hypersomnia, poor concentrating ability and poor short-term memory) (3) symptoms of impaired hormone function (decreased libido, impotence, acne, PMS, menstrual cramps, and any type of abnormal menstrual flow) (4) intolerance to chemicals (odors, foods, drugs).

Finally, joint and muscle pains (usually diagnosed "fibrositis" or "myositis") and conventional allergy symptoms (allergic rhinitis, bronchial asthma, chronic urticaria, migraine headaches, etc.) may or may not be present. These latter symptoms, while less useful in defining this syndrome, frequently prove to have been related to yeast when they clear concomitantly with disappearance of the above characteristic symptoms.

These general symptoms occur in various combinations from patient to patient and in a given patient at different times, in association with chronic superficial yeast infections predominantly in the vagina and GI tract. This combination of general and local symptoms permits definition and recognition of this condition.

Therapeutic Trial

It was observations by patients of the disappearance of these general complaints, as superficial yeast infections were brought under control, that allowed recognition of the various individual symptoms and led to the defining of this syndrome (2). It is this very same simultaneous improvement of local and general symptoms that allows the diagnosis to be confirmed after a brief (six-week) therapeutic trial of nystatin and diet.

A much longer period of treatment (usually a minimum of 2-3 years) is necessary, however, to restore immunologic competence to the point that relapse will not occur when treatment is discontinued (16). Chronic infections represent a temporary impairment of immunologic control of a particular microorganism. Thus, there must exist some degree of "immunologic tolerance" (paralysis, unresponsiveness) to the infecting organism. A chronic infection, by the very fact of its existence, reveals that such tolerance is present, even though laboratory methods may as yet be insufficiently sophisticated to demonstrate what nature is telling us. Restoration of normal immunologic control is the ultimate goal of treatment in this, as in all chronic infections.

Limitations of Laboratory Diagnosis of Chronic Yeast Infections. Even in its most severe and often fatal form—deep (systemic) candidiasis—diagnosis is largely clinical. Antibody levels frequently fail to reflect the widespread autopsy-proven dissemination of yeast into internal organs, both false positive and false negative results occurring (5). Also, blood cultures may remain negative until the moment of death, as illustrated by two reported cases of autopsy-proven, multiple-organ infection in which blood cultures were negative on 26 and 22 attempts respectively, the latter in the last 2 weeks of life (34). Until diagnostic techniques can be improved, the current situation is best described in the summation of the 1978 UCLA Conference on "Severe Candidal Infections" (35), in which it was stressed that the diagnosis of systemic candidiasis is largely one of bedside evaluation that depends on the physician's knowledge of the manifestations of the disseminated disease.

This being true for this most advanced form of candidiasis, it would seem unlikely that laboratory findings would prove any more specific or helpful in the diagnosis of the superficial form of candidiasis, or of the superficial candidiasis syndrome. The above statement, that diagnosis of deep candidiasis is largely one of bedside evaluation, could just as well have been written for the superficial candidiasis syndrome.

The unreliability of cultures in the diagnosis of superficial candidiasis was in fact demonstrated in the UAB study. Two different culture techniques were used, despite which positive vaginal cultures for yeast were reported in only 7 of 40 patients before treatment (25). Yet the first, and essential, criterion used in the selection of these patients was that there be a history of chronic yeast vaginitis, either continuous or at frequent intervals, the diagnosis of which by their personal physicians had been confirmed by temporary improvement of vaginal symptoms with anti-yeast vaginal therapy. In the UAB study, if diagnosis had been based on culture rather than on clinical symptoms, in only 7 of the women would the vaginitis have been treated. Yet improvement in vaginal symptoms was reported significant at $P<.001$ (25). Improvement was reported by 36 of the 40 women!

The difficulty of culturing yeast in deep as well as in superficial candidiasis suggests that perhaps more appropriate culture media are needed for this particular state of virulence of C. albicans. If we treat only when cultures are positive, many patients with systemic candidiasis will die, and those with the superficial candidiasis syndrome will remain untreated, only to continue their fruitless and expensive search for an answer to their chronic health problems.

Candida infections continue to be aggravated, often for years, by the repeated use and *mis-use* of antibiotics, contraceptive hormones, and steroids that are employed to treat the infections, hormone problems, allergies, muscle and joint complaints, etc. that so uniformly characterize this condition. At truly staggering cost, specialists in many fields conscientiously investigate these individual complaints with radiologic, endoscopic, and laboratory procedures. This happens, not once, but repeatedly in an illness that may span many years and that almost always is considered psychoneurosis, only because such extensive (and expensive) testing fails to yield evidence of organic illness.

A simple alternative is to suspect the cause by a careful history of the symptoms—their nature, sequence, and whether aggravated by antibiotics etc. and to verify or reject the tentative diagnosis of "superficial candidiasis syndrome" by a brief six-week (or less) therapeutic trial of nystatin and proper diet, accompanied to the extent possible by avoidance of those factors that led to the problem in the first place. The use in this way of this safe and relatively inexpensive drug can establish the correct diagnosis, lead to major relief of symptoms, and prevent the continued expenditure of unbelievably large amounts of money on tests searching for that which is not present and on drugs that poorly alleviate the symptoms, many of which (antibiotics, contraceptive hormones, corticosteroids) indeed often aggravate and perpetuate the illness. The diagnosis is verified in 6 weeks or less when symptoms show marked improvement, or disappear entirely.

We can look forward to the availability of a laboratory test that will determine conclusively when yeast is the cause of the general symptoms—a test that will determine whether a fungus that is universally present in humans is causing generalized symptoms, in addition to the accepted local manifestations. Such a test is not available, either for deep (systemic) or superfical candidiasis. Meanwhile, careful clinical evaluation followed by a brief therapeutic trial is necessary to identify subjects whose symptoms are caused by this yeast. In an on-going search for a diagnostic test, a number of abnormalities have been found, some of which have been reported (18).

Summary

Full treatment with oral and vaginal nystatin, diet and immunotherapy resulted in clearing of the generalized symptoms described by women with yeast vaginitis—symptoms that had proved to be highly resistant to treatment with vaginal anti-yeast drugs.

Partial treatment with nystatin alone, the dose of which changed each 8 weeks as it was replaced partially or completely with oral and vaginal placebo, resulted in improvement in general symptoms that coincided with improvement in the vaginal yeast infections. Five different statistical analyses of the UAB data demonstrated the statistical significance of the relationship between these generalized symptoms and those originating at the sites of mucosal infection by yeast:

(1) By linear trend: (Figs. 5A & 5B). The greater the total amount of oral and vaginal nystatin received, the greater the improvement in *both* the 15 non-vaginal symptoms and in the 9 psychological measures, $P<.03$ and $P<.01$, respectively.

(2) By exact probability: (Figs. 2B & 2C). Twenty-four of the 25 generalized symptoms improved during the 32 weeks of nystatin/placebo treatment, significantly non-random, $P<.0000008$.

(3) By ANOVA: ANOVA over 32 weeks (Fig. 4) was significant (26), $P<.05$.

(4) By meta-analysis: Meta-analysis, combining the two halves of the study (26), was significant, $P<.01$.

(5) By Student's *t* test: (Fig. 4). When the 40 subjects were compared in two groups—high vs low-dose nystatin—significance was found for improvement in those on high-dose for the first 16 weeks of the 32-week study, $P<.03$. Powerfully replicating this finding was the fact that the group who for the second 16 weeks changed from high-dose to low-dose nystatin immediately became worse, while those now on high-dose immediately became better. At week 20 the difference was significant, $P<.05$. Both changes persisted until the end of 32 weeks.

This reversal of symptoms in *each* group eliminates placebo effect as the alternative explanation for the improvement in generalized symptoms, since placebo effect could not cause patients to become both better and worse.

Partial treatment in the blinded UAB study led to partial improvement. Full treatment in the present study led to essentially complete elimination of symptoms.

Conclusions

(1) Chronic superficial yeast infections may lead to generalized symptoms.

(2) A 6-week therapeutic trial of nystatin and diet is adequate to establish or reject the diagnosis of this, the "superficial candidiasis syndrome". This simple, safe and relatively inexpensive six-week therapeutic trial will identify yeast as the cause of this complex of symptoms and stop the very large expense entailed in the repeated investigation of these symptoms.

(3) Symptoms used to define the "chronic fatigue syndrome" closely parallel those first reported (2) in association with chronic superficial yeast infections, and have been found to be relieved by the anti-yeast drugs nystatin and ketoconazole, each administered together with a low carbohydrate-low yeast diet.

(4) We in the medical profession, by the widespread use *and misuse* of antibiotics, progesterone, and immunosuppressant therapy, are inducing but not adequately treating chronic superficial yeast infections of the gastrointestinal tract and vagina. The chronic generalized symptoms that may result are almost always then attributed to psychoneurosis following repetitive testing, resulting in treatment that is symptomatic rather than treatment that is directed at the cause of the illness. The drugs used to treat the symptoms often include antibiotics, contraceptive hormones, and immunosuppressants—therapies that in fact aggravate and perpetuate the chronic superficial candidiasis syndrome.

(5) These results show that the proper design of a study to evaluate this condition is a between-subjects comparison of oral and vaginal nystatin to oral and vaginal placebo. Six to eight weeks is adequate for such a between-subjects comparison.

Acknowledgment

The Critical Illness Research Foundation was formed in 1982 by Mr. and Mrs. Emil Hess. We are deeply indebted to them for making possible this study as well as the continuing laboratory investigation of the superficial candidiasis syndrome.

References

1. Odds FC. Candida and candidosis. Leicester: Leicester University Press; 1979: 249.
2. Truss CO. Tissue injury induced by candida albicans: mental and neurologic manifestations. J Orthomolecular Psychiatry 1978; 7:17-37
3. Harvard Medical School Health Letter. Yeast: Raising Questions. Feb. 1987; 12, No 4:1-3
4. Anderson JA, Chas H, Claman HN, et al. Candidiasis hypersensitivity syndrome J Allergy Clin Immunol 1986; 78: 271-3
5. Odds FC. Candida and candidosis. 2nd Ed. London, Bailliere Tindall; 1988: 233-234
6. Council on scientific affairs. JAMA 1987; 258: 1507
7. Shapiro GG, Anderson JA. Commentary. Pediat 1988; 82:6:936
8. University of California, Berkeley. Wellness Letter 1987; 3:8
9. Blonz ER. "Is there an epidemic of chronic candidiasis in our midst?" JAMA 1986; 256:3138-3139
10. Candidiasis: Current misconceptions: Infectious diseases and immunization committee; Canad Med Assoc J. 1988; 139: 728-730
11. FDA Consumer Bulletin. October 1989; p.29
12. Truss CO. Restoration of immunologic competence to Candida albicans. J Orthomolecular Psychiatry 1980; 9: 287-301
13. Yeast-Human Interaction Conference. Birmingham, Alabama Gesell Institute and Critical Illness Research Foundation, December 9-11, 1983
14. Yeast-Human Interaction Conference. San Francisco, CA Gesell Institute and Critical Illness Research Foundation, March 29-31, 1985
15. Crook WG. The yeast connection. 3rd ed. Jackson, Tenn; Professional Books, 1989
16. Truss CO. The Missing diagnosis, 2nd Ed. Birminghan, AL. The Missing Diagnosis, Inc. 1986
17. Truss CO. The role of Candida albicans in human illness. J Orthomolecular Psychiatry 1981; 10: 228-238
18. Truss CO. Metabolic abnormalities in patients with chronic candidiasis: the acetaldehyde hypothesis. J Orthomolecular Psychiatry 1984; 13: 66-93
19. Axelsen NH. Analysis of human Candida precipitins by quantititative immunoelectrophoresis. Scan J Immunol 1976; 5: 177-90
20. Iwata K. Fungal toxins as a parasitic factor responsible for the establishment of fungal infections. Mycopathologia 1978; 65:141-154
21. Louria DB. Candida infections in experimental animals. In: Candidiasis, ed. Bodey GP, Fainstein V. New York: Raven Press, 1985: 46-47
22. Cutler JE, Friedman L, Milner KC. Biological and chemical characterization of toxic substances from Candida albicans. Infect Immun 1972; 6: 616-627
23. Van Niel CB, Anderson EH. On the occurrence of fermentative assimilation. J Cell and Comp Physiol 1941; 17:49-56
24. Bernard EM, Christiansen KJ, et al. Rate of arabinitol production by pathogenic yeast. J Clin Microbiol 1981; 14: 189-194.
25. Dismukes WE, Wade JS, et al. A randomized double-blind trial of nystatin therapy for the candidiasis hypersensitivity syndrome. N Engl J Med 1990; 323:25: 1717-1722.
26. Truss CO, Truss CV, Cutler RB, Llabre M. A controlled trial of nystatin for the candidiasis hypersensitivity syndrome. N Engl J Med 1991; 324:22:1592-1593
27. Wade JC, Schimpff SC, et al. A comparison of trimethoprim-sulfamethoxazole plus nystatin with gentamicin plus nystatin in the prevention of infections in acute leukemia. N. Engl J Med 1981; 304: 1057-1062

28. Wechsler D: Manual for Wechsler adult intelligence scale-revised. Psychological Corporation. Harcourt Brace, Jovanovich N.Y. 1981
29. Meyers JL. Fundamentals of experimental design, 3rd ed., Boston, MA Allyn and Bacon, 1979; 431-2
30. Crandall M. Allergic predisposition in recurrent vulvo-vaginal candidiasis. J Adv Med 1991; 4:21-38
31. Holmes GP, Kaplan JE, Gantz NM, et al. Chronic fatigue syndrome: a working case definition. Ann Int Med 1988; 108:387-389
32. Jessop C. Chronic fatigue syndrome conference. Chronic Fatigue Syndrome Quarterly, April 15, 1989 San Francisco, California
33. Bennett J. Searching for the yeast connection (editorial). N Engl J Med 1990; 323: 25:1766-1767
34. Bodey GP, Fainstein V. Systemic candidiasis. In: Candidiasis, ed Bodey, GP. and Fainstein, V. New York. Raven Press, 1985; 147-148
35. Edwards JE Jr. Summary. in Edwards JE Jr (moderator) Severe candidal infections. Clinical prespective, immune defense mechanisms, and current concepts in therapy. Ann Int Med 1978; 89:103

Reprinted previously in *The Missing Diagnosis*

1) Truss, C. O.: Tissue Injury Induced by Candida Albicans: Mental and Neurologic Manifestations. Journal of Orthomolecular Psychiatry 1978; 7: 17–37

2) Truss, C. O.: Restoration of Immunologic Competence to Candida Albicans. Journal of Orthomolecular Psychiatry 1980; 9: 287–301

3) Truss, C. O.: The Role of Candida Albicans in Human Illness. Journal of Orthomolecular Psychiatry 1981; 10: 228–238